On the Way to Walking

The Essential Guide to
Natural Movement Development ™

Lenore Grubinger, RSMT, IDME, CST

Amajoy ™

Developmental
Movement & Bodywork

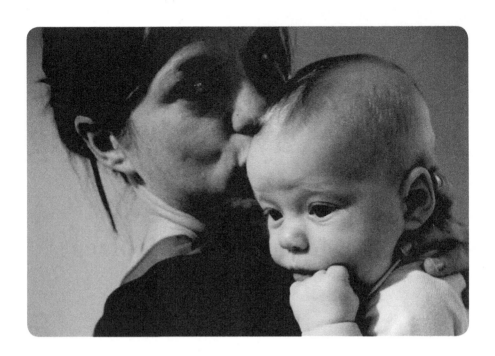

Published by Amajoy™ Developmental Movement and Bodywork
150 Nonotuck Street Florence, MA 01062-1908

Book Design by Jahara Sara Conz and Lenore Grubinger

First Printing, April 2016
ISBN 978-0-692-68635-5

Dedicated to babies, parents, and caretakers the world over

Nothing in this book is as important as the love between you

Dear Reader,

If possible, read this book close to your baby's arrival time so that you have a glimpse of how he or she will learn to move, once born.

If you are reading when Baby is already here, start in the section that feels most relevant and then refer back.

For Grandparents, please bring this book on your next visit to your sweetie. Try to get on the floor, or pull a low chair close to Baby's floor-play space, and have fun.

Please note that the use of "he" and "she" pronouns varies by chapter.

Make a small group at home, or join our online community. The practices go better with friends —for you and Baby.

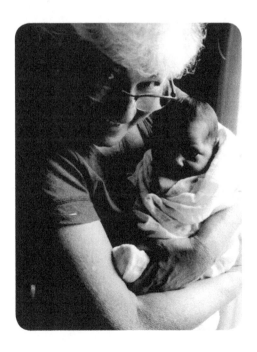

Table of Contents

Appendices

My Hopes

To help parents and providers:

- Understand and use Natural Movement Development as a lifestyle aid for the health of your whole family.

- Be a *flexion teacher** for Baby.

- Engage Baby's *reflex responses** by providing Baby with positions that are alternatives to propping.

- Recognize and respect Baby's rhythms, intentions, and communications.

- Alleviate Baby's digestive discomfort and other stress by practicing your variations of *Baby Ball* as her home base.

- Help Baby rest and move on her less familiar side during caretaking and play to protect and enhance her bilateral development.

- Choose products that support, rather than inhibit, Natural Movement Development. Make your home a safe, sensory-rich place to play that gives the whole family opportunities to move.

- Include Baby's movement play in families' choices for sustainability.

- Let go of shoulds in relation to the practices, and find your own way. If a practice is difficult, please consider a lesson with a developmental movement specialist.

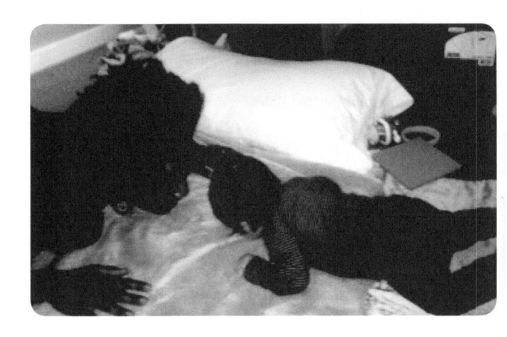

On the Way to Walking

An Overview

This book is for babies and their parents. It is for well babies. It is also for babies who had special stress at birth and after. And it can help inform programs for those with special needs. The principles and practices apply to all infants, yet vary with each individual.

The most frequent remark I hear from parents in over thirty years of serving families is that they wish they had started Natural Movement Development sooner. They say they wish they had known these practices at the beginning of Baby's life. I hope this book fulfills that wish.

Time lines are not provided and months are rarely indicated because we are focused on what Baby is doing more than on when she does it.

If Baby grows up with *Natural Movement Development** she'll enjoy long weeks of TummyTime play, lots of belly-crawling, and kneeling at your lap while learning to crawl on hands-and-knees. Once standing, Baby will enjoy another period of side-stepping before she begins walking. I will highlight these foundational natural movements Baby makes to help you aid her development to be healthy and comfortable.

In the first section, you will find a pictorial overview of **Natural Movement Development**. It is there to refer to as you hold, care for, and move with Baby from birth to walking.

In **Foundational Early Months**, you will find support for your new life with Baby at home.

Baby will be spending a lot of time eating, sleeping, and being in your arms. This is a once-in-a-lifetime period for Baby and you. We'll observe and meet Baby where she is, and she will be the focus of our days. This is a foundational, moment-savoring time for the whole family.

In **The TummyTime Lifestyle** we'll go over the things that families have found bring ease in TummyTime. I'll help you protect that precious floor-time in the early months because I have seen that it contributes to Baby's healthy brain and body development. TummyTime, like Early InnerTime, gives Baby a positive foundation.

In **Starting to Get Around,** we'll stick together as Baby makes her big shift to moving about. In this period, she transitions from total physical dependence on you, to some interdependent movements with you, and some independent movements of her own, beyond TummyTime.

Finally, in **Busy, Busy,** we will get to know this amazing, active, curious, and vocal person who was recently your tiny baby. We'll savor this next special time—the one before walking—during which Baby develops capacity and confidence to move in your safe, sensory-rich home.

Key to Symbols

It's All Connected

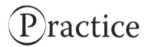

Focus Points

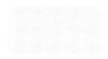ractice

Methods of Holding, Moving, and Relating with Baby

Leads to:

Highlights What Comes Next

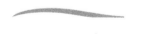

Try It Yourself

Natural Movement Alternatives

Taking Care Along the Way

* Asterisks indicate further explanation in the glossary

On the Way to Walking

Natural Movement Development

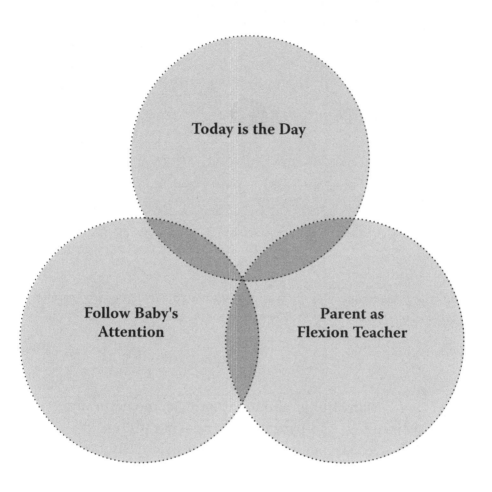

Today is the Day

Follow Baby's Attention

Parent as Flexion Teacher

What is this family doing?

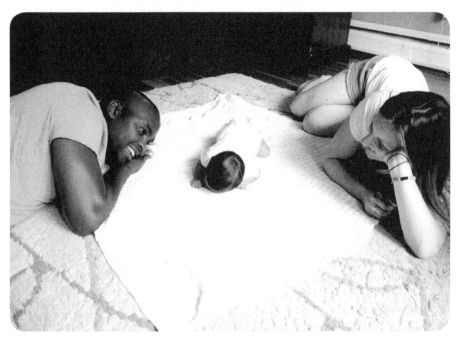

After the long pregnancy, the intensity of birth, and the building of new routines at home, this family relaxes in TummyTime for the first time.

" Many things about parenting come naturally. My intuition as a parent is essential but it's not exclusive. My son was born with restrictive tightness on one side of his neck and body and we sought out some help for him. I found that Natural Movement Development allowed me to combine gentle practices while supporting my intuition and my child. "

A Mother

1. Natural Movement Development

Welcome! You are on a remarkable journey—the extraordinary, and ordinary, adventure of parenting.

Both confidence and uncertainty are present; thoughts swirl throughout the day from amazement to concern. Will Baby be okay? Should I follow Baby or should I teach her something? Isn't she fine the way that she is? Can I make a mistake? What should I do? What's the balance between nurture and nature?

Together we will address these questions so that you can care for Baby with more trust in your intuition, more capacity to relate with Baby as a fully-feeling, three-dimensionally moving person, and more confidence in your ability to parent.

Let's think for a moment of Baby as a growing plant. This plant starts as a seed in soil full of the nutrients it needs to develop a good root system for a strong stem which can then support the buds and flowers that follow. We will explore natural ways to help Baby grow so that her development is well and appropriately fertilized, planted in your arms and then growing from the floor up without you doing too much or too little. You'll enjoy watching Baby's every new movement with the eagerness of an avid gardener.

This book emphasizes letting Baby grow in her own time instead of pulling on her stem to make her flowers emerge. I'll show you how you can help by moving her at her existing skill level so you don't put her ahead of what she can do herself. I'll share practices that give Baby the most natural route to safe, skillful, independent movement, from bud to flower. This requires learning for you at first, yet it becomes easy and can simplify parenting over time, allowing more enjoyment for Baby and you.

I call this Natural Movement Development™. We wait, observe, and assist each child in all the stages leading up to, and including, standing and walking. We hold Baby curled in our arms, we lay her down, and lean her against us. Later, we help her crawl on her belly, then on her hands-and-knees, to kneel in our laps. Until Baby can stand on her own, we mostly refrain from holding her in a standing position, or putting her in equipment which maintains her in sitting or standing. This holding or placing of Baby in dependent, upright positions is called *propping**.

Propping has become common in two decades time; products that prop Baby dominate the infant marketplace. Specifically, equipment which maintains Baby in sitting, standing, and jumping positions has become a routine part of the things parents are expected to use for Baby. Propping babies into positions they can not achieve themselves, as a lifestyle, can inhibit independent movement or result in difficulties with coordination, learning, and sensory processing.

The propping lifestyle is problematic because it prevents opportunities for some of Baby's reflexes to respond in the way that nature intends. These are the very ones Baby needs in order to achieve upright positions independently.

In recent years, the American Medical Association (AMA) has declared that TummyTime is also important. Pediatricians now say "back to sleep, prone for play" and recommend twenty minutes a day on the belly for Baby. Some parents fear the tummy position for their babies due to its association with Sudden Infant Death Syndrome (SIDS) during sleep and do not follow the "prone for play" recommendation, despite it being for Baby's awake times. Products that address this anxiety by maintaining Baby in upright positions have been filling homes ever since.

Back-sleeping for infants, parents' fear of TummyTime, Baby's unfamiliarity with this position, along with ever-present propping, have altered infant development. Fewer babies crawl and more go directly to walking than ever before.

I don't think this is anyone's fault, especially not parents'. Rather it is the result of a marketplace reflecting—and generating—an uncontested emphasis on accelerated development, with a high value on growing up, and upright, as soon as possible.

Parents are considered "good" when they buy "good" things for their kids, particularly things which support this falsely prized verticality. I am here to help you focus your lens of sustainable living on Baby's body, brain, and movement, his communications, and your physical relationship. This framework for sustainability with Baby includes your body, your intuition, and your home as "good" things.
The best, actually.

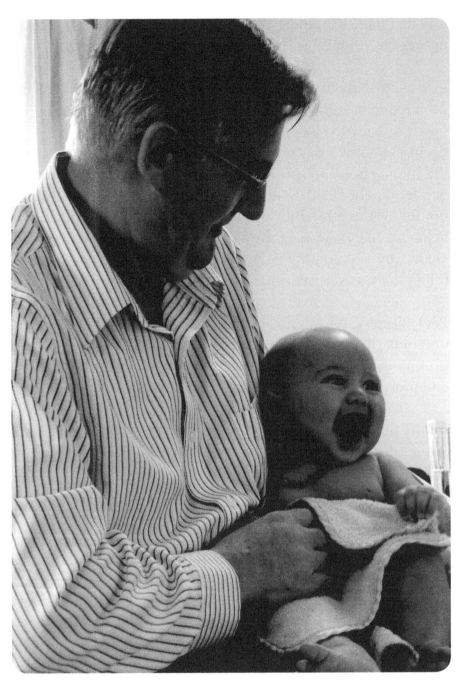

Grandpa and grandson, what a joy!

We'll explore how to use natural, prop-free positions for caretaking and play. I'll provide you with alternatives to the propping lifestyle that is all around you. I aim to help you trust your intuition and your Baby's communications.

These positions are methods to be used when you are picking Baby up or putting her down, and for when you are playing. Natural positions are those which Baby can achieve independently and from which she can move safely. They prepare her for her next gain in movement skills, perception, *self-regulation**, and communication.

We're not here to 'make Baby better.' How could we possibly, when she is already so amazingly, indescribably, and deliciously perfect? We're here to make things easier, more comfortable, and more sustainable for our families.

Natural Movement Development™ is for both well babies and challenged babies. A well baby, whether she has been propped or not, benefits from Natural Movement Development™. It is also appropriate for the following:

- *low tone** or *high tone**.
- genetic or neurological syndromes.
- digestive discomfort or disorder.
- effects of trauma that occurred *in utero* or during birth.
- low or high weight at birth or in infancy.
- early birth, late, breech, or Cesarean.
- strong arching of the back and thrusting of the legs
- sleep disruption

Why practice Natural Movement Development? Would it be more natural not to? You may think so, yet as parents, we are always making choices as we hold, move, and position Baby. We have practices about how we spend our day with baby, what we do and don't buy for Baby, and activities we choose or avoid. Our parenting day is full of belief-driven practices, many of them outside of awareness. Several of these practices are cultural habits regarding keeping Baby upright to comfort her and teach her to move.

In my practice at Amajoy Developmental Movement and Bodywork I use Natural Movement Development to bring awareness to Baby's current movement choices and provide Baby, and you, with new options. These options are based on what Baby will learn to do on her own utilizing the reflex resources that are built into her system.

I am here to help you grow Baby's movement from the floor up, to gently bring more floor-play into your life if you have already been propping. While the practices require awareness at first, they become an easier, familiar part of your teamwork, and they are fun.

When we practice Natural Movement Development with Baby from birth we are helping her in the time that her reflexes are meant to engage. Whether Baby is newborn or several months old, from the point of view of her brain and body, the time to begin these practices is today.

Reflexes

Reflexes are experience-expectant pathways in every person. They determine our body's relationship to gravity, and our orientation in space. Reflexes also process and make sensations and movements.

Support for Baby's Natural Movement Development lies in moving her through the simplest, safest movements that she would do herself if she could. These are movements such as rolling off her tummy when she wants to, pushing up from her tummy as she gets a bit bigger, then moving herself through space on her tummy toward her interests.

These movements are self-fulfilling as each reflex response provides needed stimulation for other reflex responses, those that nature is ready to engage at each stage.

Reflexes, together with her attention, are a big part of what you see your new Baby doing. Reflexes require stimulation and experience to "wake up." These responses are the foundation of her later intentional movements. Baby does not have an intellectual idea to move, rather she goes towards or away from something because of interest. This is her drive to connect or protect, not a decision to exercise!

(P)ractice

Startle and Recovery

Startle and recovery is a set of reflex responses that I feel is essential for parents and providers to understand so they can provide Baby with the support she needs to fulfill these responses comfortably.

It is natural for Baby to startle and recover. This is a reflex we all have throughout our lives; it is a series of movements, not a single response. It is called the *Startle Reflex** or *Moro Reflex** and is there from birth. Startle and recovery is a whole body reflex response, engaged when Baby feels her head dropping back behind her spine.

In this whole body response, if Baby's head tips back unexpectedly or quickly, her arms thrust out, her back arches, and she cries or frowns. Then she folds back into herself, moving her head, arms, and legs together, and rests after crying. (See pgs. 101-103 for more.)

Once Baby arches back, she needs a grown-up to help her complete the full reflex response including recovering by moving her limbs toward her middle and resting. Once you notice easily when Baby startles, you can assist her to complete her recovery response. Wait until she finishes arching her body, then hold her against you so that she folds into you as you fold around her, and rest there until she is ready to move again. (See more flexion-to-flexion on pg. 64.)

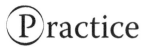ractice

Less Startling

We try to hold and move Baby so as to cause as little startling as possible. Most babies startle easily at first. It can take time and teamwork to fine-tune for less startle. There will still be some startle, especially in response to loud sounds. We aim for less startle during caretaking and play.

The essence of less startling lies in keeping Baby's neck bent slightly forward of her spine. To do so, you will need to explore what works for your body as you pick up or lower Baby. She will still startle. This is not bad for her. By observing how and when Baby startles, she shows you right where she needs your help to prevent this from occurring when you can.

Place one hand on the back of her head and neck, and your other under her behind. Keep her spine in a consistent position as you move her. This way, her head can't drop back and she doesn't have to startle unnecessarily.

Frequent unnecessary startling causes stronger muscles on the back of the body than front. This imbalance in muscle tone can in turn create vulnerability to discomfort and challenges for Baby later, both physically and emotionally.

When Baby startles, we startle too. It can be subtle, yet it affects our equilibrium. The practices of preventing startle when possible, along with helping Baby recover from startle as we help ourselves soften after startling, are at the heart of what we hope will be lifelong stress-management skills for Baby and you, individually and as a team.

What is Propping?

Propping means placing Baby into positions she can't achieve on her own. They are positions "ahead" of her existing skills and strength. From a propped position Baby doesn't yet have the skills to protect herself by putting her arms out if she tips or falls.

From the beginning, parents may be encouraged to sit Baby, and to place her over a nursing pillow or rolled towel for TummyTime. Ironically this can make it difficult for Baby to develop strength and comfort in TummyTime, and in all coordinated movement sequences other than thrusting her legs.

Early propped sitting is seen as beneficial, just as holding Baby in standing is seen as cute and helpful. These commmonplace propping practices, done with loving intention, along with the daily use of equipment that props Baby up, dominate contemporary physical experiences of infancy.

Natural Movement Development encourages you to express your care and respect for Baby physically by placing her in safe positions that she can move out of, if she wants, by way of a *safe small fall* such as a roll, without startling or tipping back.

"My Baby Loves To Stand"

Prop-standing is done with love and is well-intentioned. It can comfort Baby; if Baby gets really used to it, it is sometimes one of the only things that comforts her. Every baby has the drive to get up and get going. Standing may feel exciting when you place her there, and, if everyone lights up while she is there, she will too.

As previously stated, every time you prop-stand Baby, you strengthen reflexes in her whole body that make her push her feet out and throw her head back. Baby is not actually standing; she is balancing on her feet while you hold her up. If you let go, she would fall backwards and hit her head.

When moving naturally, Baby first "stands" on her forearms, then in a triangle shape, and then on long arms like a cobra. Next, she stands on her hands-and-knees like a table, then she stands on her knees, known as kneeling, and finally she stands on her feet independently when she is ready.

Prop-standing is loving teamwork, and can be exciting for Baby and parents. The trouble with prop-standing and prop-walking is that Baby cannot walk without the adult. She loses natural opportunities to develop her strength, balance, and coordination that precede walking. She also misses out on the leg-aligning and ankle-straightening reflexes, as well as protective responses, that are engaged by hands-and-knees-crawling. And she becomes dependent on an adult to move, at the very time that nature is trying to help her move independently.

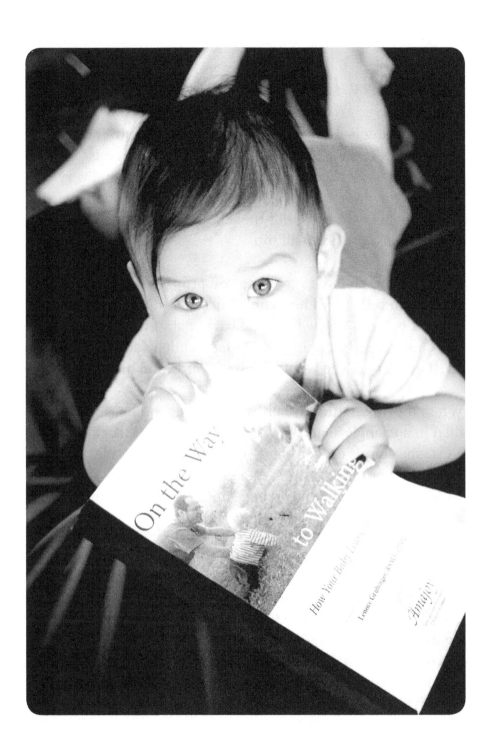

Less Propping

If you are already propping Baby occasionally, please don't feel bad or concerned. There is lots of love expressed in propping. I will show you ways to gently decrease propping and add alternative positions that you and Baby can come to know and enjoy.

Once you are propping less, Baby will expect it less. It will become second nature for both of you to choose the alternatives that you and Baby have practiced (refer to appendix 7).

Still, there may be moments when propping is needed, such as to protect your back, to keep Baby safe if you're in a rush, and those unexpected moments when you need to concentrate on something immediate.

Ironically, the emphasis on early upright positioning tends to reassure parents. It leads to the false impression that Baby is smart, even advanced, because she is upright like grown-ups. Of course you want Baby to stand and walk. I do too. I hope this book will enhance your understanding of what Baby does naturally during her time prior to standing and walking, because that time is the foundation for all her further movement. She'll have a lifetime of standing and walking, and that begins soon enough.

First, Baby has some essential moving to do on the floor. Like enjoying the time when buds ripen and open, you can enjoy the pre-walking months more if you bear in mind that this essential foundational time is short and provides important experiences for her later flowering into upright movement.

> ❝ I was walking in the park and saw a group of professional nannies socializing together. Each nanny stood by a stroller where one or two, or even three, infants were lying on their backs under a blanket, under a seat belt, with the canopy up. The nannies were chatting, texting, and snacking. After a while a couple of them left, and then the group dispersed. Each employer would later be glad to hear that her baby had been to the park. No one in the situation is concerned that the children are not moving. ❞

An Observer On her Way

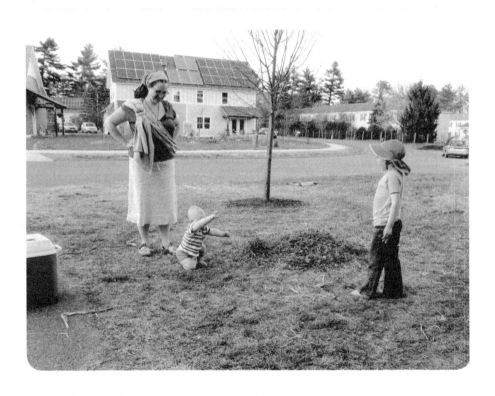

Let Baby Move

When families don't find comfortable TummyTime, Baby is typically placed into propped-sitting positions from early on. Or, Baby is contained in standing equipment, with little or no movement, along with a lot of close stimulation. Or she may be hung in a jumper by her crotch, where she pushes into her feet for long stretches.

Without our awareness of Baby's need for movement, she may spend hours each day in these passive vertical positions, and little time in free movement.

The car seat, the activity center, the harness, and even the stroller all restrict Baby's movement. When Baby is strapped in for long periods, she lies or sits and cannot move, with a limited view of what's around her. It is easy to think this equipment is beneficial, because we are reassured when we see Baby upright. And it certainly provides our busy, busy lives with a spot of appreciated babysitting.

Natural Movement Development is a commitment to teamwork for Baby and you. It includes planning your time and physical space with respect for Baby's needs as a moving individual.

"Thinking begins in movement and the senses. Baby's movement adventures are the beginning of problem solving. His active engagement in the mastery of new skills strengthens his attentive concentration. By understanding the pieces of Baby's movement development, you will come to appreciate and value his thought processes." (Chutroo B. and Jamrog S., Unpublished Manuscript)

When I had my first child, I sat and prop-stood her. I walked her by standing behind her, holding her hands, so her back arched; she hung on my hands as she moved. Once I did it, she wanted me to do it all the time. She screamed if I wouldn't walk her. When I had my second child, I never prop-sat or prop-walked him. It was awesome to see him crawl for so many months, then pull up, stand, side-step, and walk when he was ready—which was at fourteen months.

Mother of two

With my first baby, I was surprised at the competition I experienced at a couple of the mother's groups I went to. People seemed competitive about how early their baby was sitting, standing, crawling, or talking. There also was competition about the stuff people got for their kids. With my second baby, I wanted to find something less competitive. I had more confidence that hanging out with my baby was more important than measuring his milestones or buying him stuff. We went to the park, we went to the library, and we ended up with a little group that met at the cafe. It was great and I regretted what I had missed with my first child.

Mother of two

Milestones and Values Change

It's hard to recognize the style of a generation when you are living it. We live in a time of medical measuring. Much of this is beneficial; however, measuring can also stimulate worry or even fear, which can then shift some of the focus off the family bond and benefits, some of which are not as carefully measured. In particular, weight-gain relative to age is measured more often than in decades past.

In recent generations, babies actually did develop a little differently than they do today. For example, children weren't stood as often, and there wasn't a fear of placing Baby on her front. (The opposite, in fact!) An acquaintance might ask, "Boy or girl?" "What's his/her name?" "How old?" Now, along with these questions, folks ask if Baby sleeps through the night, eats well, and how much she weighs.

If you aim for simple and sustainable parenting, I hope this book helps your efforts by providing a perspective which is less measurement-oriented, less equipment-based, and more body-focused. Our attention is on Baby's skills and experiences, regardless of whether they occur early, at an average time, or are delayed. I want to help you meet Baby where she is, and help her find the next smallest possible gain, regardless of her age. I hope Baby will walk, talk, and read --just like everyone else does. For now we'll take the emphasis off of how much or how little Baby is delayed or advanced, and focus instead on what she does now and how we can increase her comfort and fertilize her growth and capability from here. Overall, we focus more on watching what Baby does and what she is trying to do than on measuring her milestones.

What's happening here?

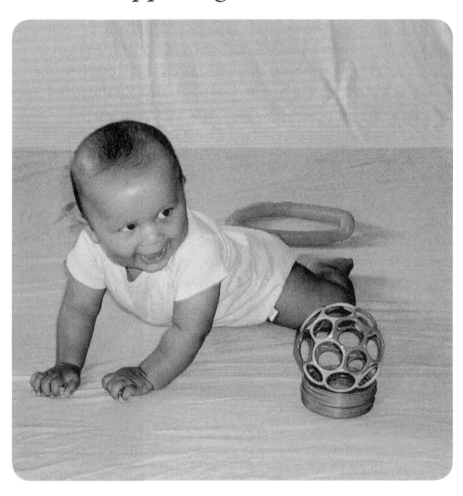

This five-and-a-half-month-old plays on his tummy. He is smiling at his Mom nearby, as he holds himself up on his arms. He is moving between Belly-Crawling and Hands-and-Knees Crawling.

Natural Movement Development Highlights These Progressions...

- Lying on all four sides before rolling.

- Rolling before belly-crawling.

- Leaning into her own side before sitting independently.

- Belly-crawling and moving into or out of sitting are overlapping skills happening in an overlapping time period.

- Belly-crawling before hands-and-knees crawling.

- Rocking on hands-and-knees before crawling on hands-and-knees.

- Hands-and-knees crawling before standing.

- Kneeling on the way to standing, and kneeling back from hands-and-knees crawling.

- Side-stepping before walking.

If Baby's movements have unfolded differently than this, that's okay! The practices are for Baby and you no matter how she is developing; every Baby goes on her way differently.

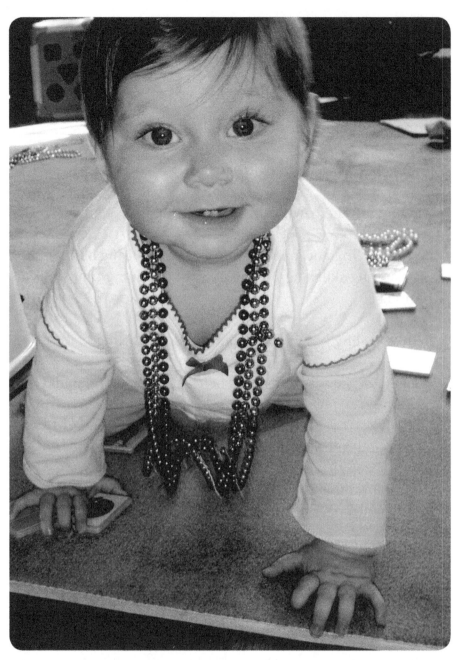

This ten-month-old girl is having fun crawling with necklaces.

If you choose Natural Movement Development for your family, you are likely to notice other parents hold and move their Baby differently than you do. At first, in social settings, Baby might seem behind others because she is lying down, while some are accustomed to being propped up in sitting.

With your support, your Baby will be happy lying and rolling, and, later, crawling and sitting on her way to walking, and so will you. She will catch up to her prop-sat and prop-stood peers on her own strong foundations. She will use her natural movement skills based on the engagement of her amazing web of reflex responses at the time they best support her development.

We usually think of reflexes as a reaction for which the pediatrician checks. Reflexes are far more meaningful than that; they animate every cell with a readiness to sense, respond, and move within the pull of gravity and in the world around. They govern every move Baby makes before she has conscious choice; they are the responses that create conscious movement.

When the reflexes emerge in their natural order, they engage and strengthen muscle groups and movement sequences that are the foundation of the next natural movement.

If I were with you in person, I would be striving to provide the gentlest possible amount of support, within Baby's interest, to trigger her reflexes to do the movements she is trying to do. I hope you will proceed in this manner, knowing that Baby does not need to be "fixed." It is natural to have some stress, and to benefit from some help. I will remind you along the way to go gently and patiently, putting love first.

Essentials On the Way to Natural Movement Development

Connect before you do anything

Take a deep breath and feel your love. Pause to enjoy Baby in her present state. If she's content, imitate what she's doing. Take time to move as she does, to feel in your body what it's like in hers.

Follow Baby's attention and interest

Bring your attention and curiosity, so that you can notice and follow Baby's interests and choices. The practices go most smoothly when you are following what Baby wants to do.

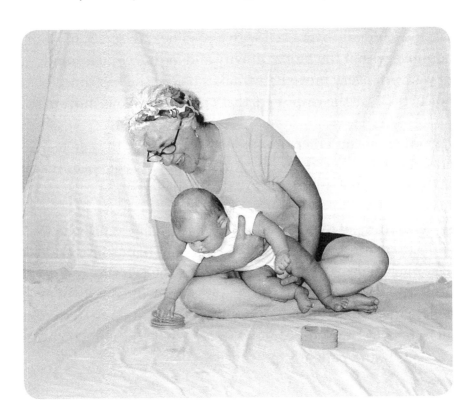

Light touch

Provide the least amount of help possible in order to let Baby do as much of the movement she can do independently. Cease practice if it feels like forcing. Try again another time.

Wait for the pauses

Practice the positions or movements with Baby during the pauses in her strong thrusts. These strong movements have a natural cycle which includes a brief pause. When Baby arches back or thrusts her legs, wait until you feel her brief softening before you move her. This takes careful attention and patience. We never have to get it right now, or even today. If it's hard, let it go. Please look for the pause another time soon.

Short and sweet

Keep practice short and sweet. Remove your hands as soon as Baby finds the new position or takes over the movement.

Rest is integration

Let Baby rest after each practice. The rest is as important as the practice. Allow recuperation through crying, nursing, playing, swaddling, or resting as needed. Listen and observe; Baby will show you when she needs to recuperate. Remember we are more goal oriented than she is. There is no rush; she learns best if we follow her rhythm of eat, learn, rest.

Brief and often

It is more important for Baby to experience a new position briefly and repeatedly than it is to stay in the position. It is beneficial for Baby to be in the new position, even if she does not stay there on her own.

It's not personal

Try not to take it personally when Baby does not want to practice. Baby is not "non-cooperative." It is a matter of reflexes and responses from her low brain.

Refrain from talking about it with Baby

Generally, refrain from talking with Baby about what you're doing. Remain playful, try making up a little tune or rhythm. "I love your sweet legs" is easier for both of you than "mommy is going to try to bend your leg."

Catch the fresh moments for movement

Try not to practice when either you or Baby are tired. Also, refrain from new movements if anyone in the family has a cold. Sometimes it takes a long time for a cold to run through a family. You might need patience while Baby's immune system does its job over days or even weeks. There is no rush. Resting and healing come first. When Baby, you, and others are well again, you can refocus on movement practice.

Honor the first time

The first try with each practice is the hardest. Sometimes Baby exclaims or cries when doing a new movement, particularly when moving on her less familiar side. Stop the practice and make her comfort your priority. Subsequent practices will likely be easier for both of you.

Decrease startle and increase recovery

Focus on holding and moving Baby so that her startle reflex doesn't engage unnecessarily; try not to let her head drop back. If this happens, take time to let her regroup in flexion by bringing her head and arms towards the front of her body before you continue.

Caretaking before movement

The practices are not things you "are supposed to do." They are things you can try when Baby's other needs are met. Some days there won't be time for movement practice. You'll be too busy attending in other ways to Baby. This is natural too. There is no rush in Natural Movement Development and no "shoulds."

Respect transitions

Transitions are part of daily life; they take time and energy. Leaving time and building skills for transitions is an essential and understated part of parenting.

From Careful Thinking to Easy Ways

At first you may be learning and thinking as you try to feel Baby move while you try a practice. After your initial conscious focus, these can become part of your day-to-day ways.

Try it yourself

Doing it yourself and noticing how it feels is called *embodiment*.* Embodiment increases understanding and empathy and makes it all more fun. Doing the movements yourself is essential to your success with this book.

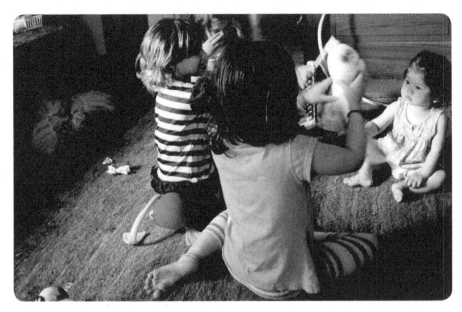

Eleven-month-old girl visits with some bigger kids.

" Teaching yoga, I am aware of the importance of connecting to the body and spending time on the floor to move. As an occupational therapy student, I was able to bring this experience of embodiment and floor-time to a classroom of first-graders. After guiding the children through yoga poses and animal movements, I invited them to their tummies on the floor to do a worksheet. The children began to quiet their voices, relax, and focus on the academic task. This reaffirmed my already existing belief that creating opportunities for children to play, rest, and work in TummyTime is important for their developing brains and bodies at every age! "

A Yoga Instructor and Occupational Therapist

For Every Body at Every Age

Natural Movement Development is not only for infants.
It is never too late to use movement helpfully for anyone.
It is best to start early because it is easiest for Baby and family
to assist reflex development when it is organically occurring;
however, the brain, the body, and the family are an open
system and the best time to start is when the chance occurs.

While infant brains grow most quickly, brain growth continues
in children, adolescents, and adults. When applied with love
and respect, movement, play, and intentional touch aid the
brain to grow and change. This remains true at every age.

Children benefit from play which draws from the practices in
this book. Parents are encouraged to join play to gain insight
into what each child chooses, and does not choose, to do.
Through this play, infants, toddlers, children, and adolescents
can increase their comfort, flexibility, and capability in body,
mind, and spirit.

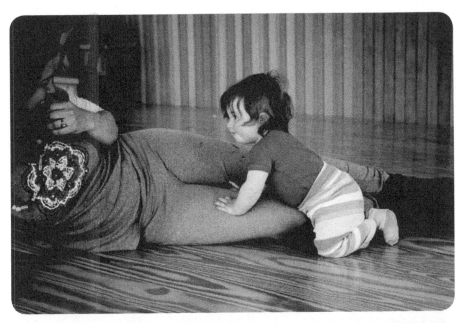

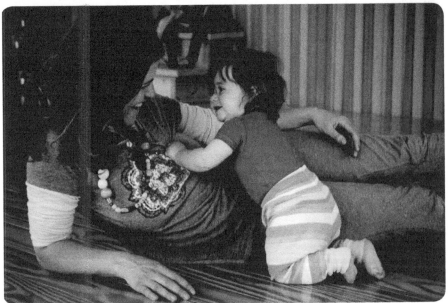

Nine-month-old girl stops by for a lap visit with Mom as she crawls around.

Natural Movement Development Your Way

This book begins with your first moments with Baby after she is born. Baby is like a seedling planted in your arms. This is where you will feed, love, and hold her with your responsive attention and care. When you are not holding her or wearing her, you can place her lying down on her back or front, left or right. You will watch her movement grow, from the floor up. She will get stronger at lifting her head and supporting herself on her forearms. Her strength will then progress down her whole body, as she learns to roll and move through space.

During these months, this book is a companion for you, and for each change on the way. It is meant to be with you on the floor, while you are with Baby.

You are invited to try the movements Baby is doing. This informs compassion, is good exercise, and Baby usually finds you entertaining!

You will likely discover pieces of your own development, such as how or if you belly-crawled, and which side of your body you use more than the other when moving from sitting to standing.

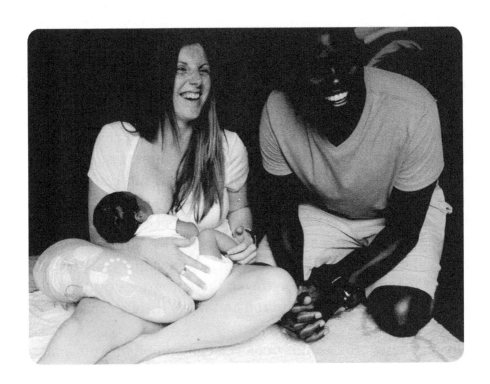

The practices engage Baby's reflexes. Reflex engagement is what makes Natural Movement Development natural. It is body-based, and will make intuitive sense. Because we are encouraged to place Baby ahead, and are not aware of some natural positions, they need to be learned—even though they are natural.

Natural Movement Development is for all families. It is for infants and children developing typically, *and* for those with extra stress and special needs. The application varies with the individual. Special needs children and their parents require more support than what this book can provide, yet the practices can aid your family.

These practices teach positions and movements that are common to all babies, yet every child and family experiences them uniquely. There is not a right or wrong way to do the practices. There is not a definitive order to development or to the practices; they are all interrelated. Most often there are several practices that are appropriate to explore during each phase of Baby's development. Some of the practices remain relevant throughout your parenting adventure.

If you feel worry, I think it is important to listen.
Do make an appointment to check in with your pediatrician. If she or he tells you that the issue that you are concerned about is something that your baby will 'grow out of,' you may be relieved. Yet, you may still feel some unease or have questions. That's the time to consult with a developmental movement professional. Having a movement lesson does not mean that there is something 'wrong' with Baby. It means that there may be reflex or sensory discomfort, or both, and you can learn how to address these to increase Baby's comfort.

Worry can at times be a reminder to seek information.
Perhaps you'll get information about your style of worrying!
If you learn about Baby's particular needs early in her life, you may save yourself more worry—and expense—by knowing what is going on with her, so you can learn to help her thrive.

A Summary of Natural Movement Development in Pictures from Birth to Standing

When allowed and supported, each baby, with her own variations, practices and progresses through the following movements. Some occur concurrently, others more sequentially. Most of the skills weave together and do not happen in a linear sequence.

Baby will likely progress from lying down to rolling. Then she might push back, and over many weeks, learn to crawl forward on her belly. From there she'll learn to push up to safe, independent sitting, then lean over to hands-and-knees crawling. Soon she'll be kneeling, then standing, side-stepping, and eventually walking on her own. Yes, the adorable, dependent small bundle who is your newborn baby will do all this in a matter of months. And he or she will keep coming back to you, on the way.

This is Natural Movement Development. It supports brain and body, child and parent.

Please refer to the summary as you and your family move through the practices.

Resting in Baby Ball

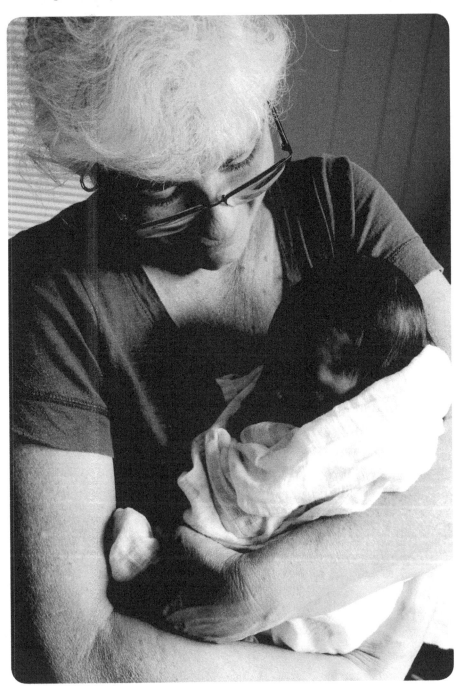

Side-lying

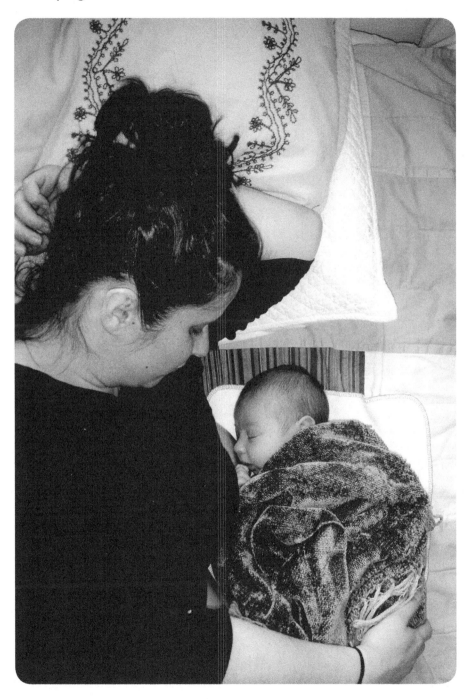

Lies comfortably on tummy, and back

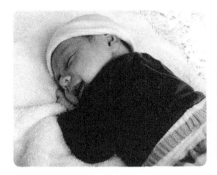 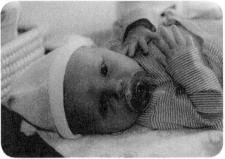

Rests comfortably on left side, right side

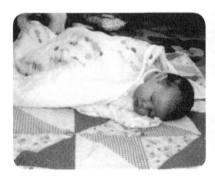 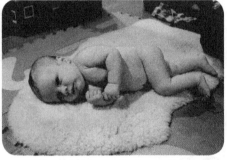

Lifts and manages head while on tummy

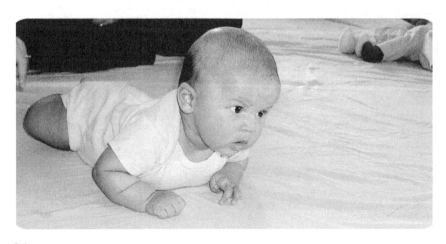

Rests on forearms

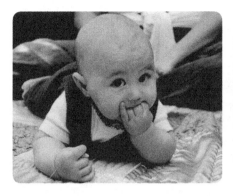
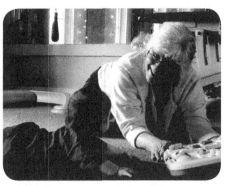

Rolls from tummy to back, back to tummy

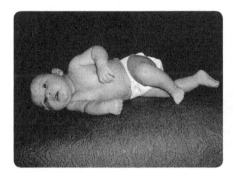
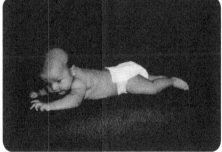

Lies comfortably on back (or backs, with twins)

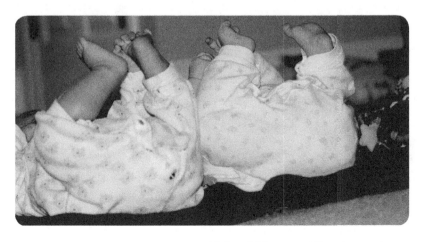

Pushes up on long strong arms

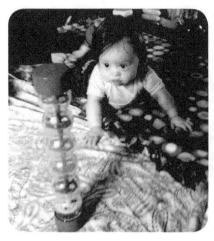 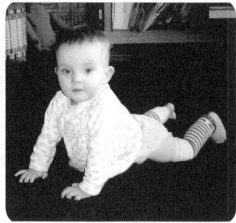

Slides backward by pushing with long arms

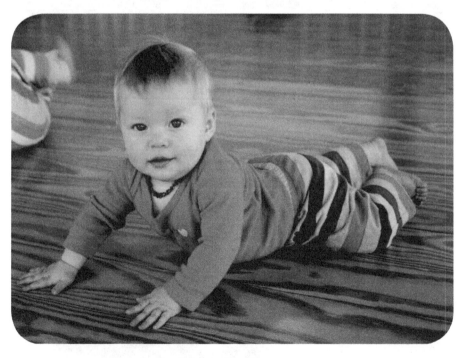

Belly-crawls forward toward something of interest

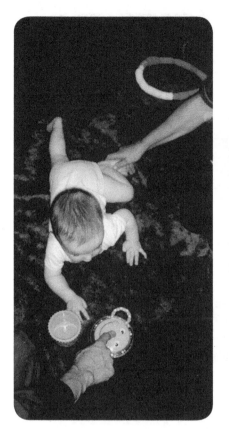
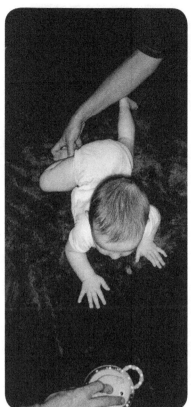

Pivots on tummy

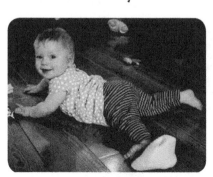
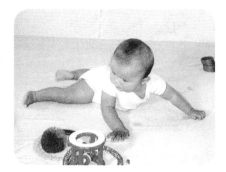

Pushes up from tummy to rock on hands-and-knees

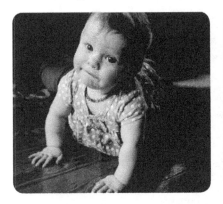 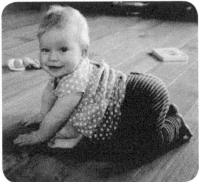

Plays and rests on purpose between side-lying and sitting

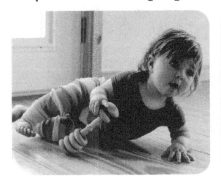 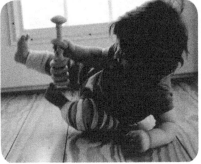

Pushes from side-leaning into sitting

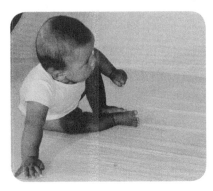 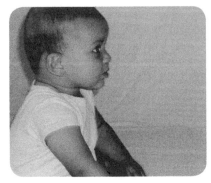

Sits hands-free with long legs or legs bent

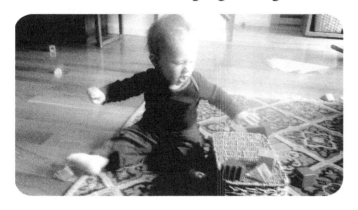

Moves from sitting down to tummy

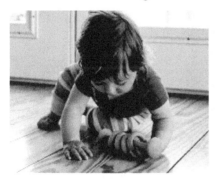 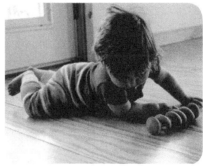

Moves from sitting onto hands-and-knees

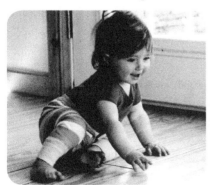 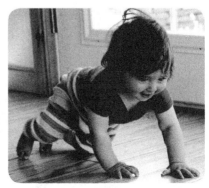

Crawls on hands-and-knees

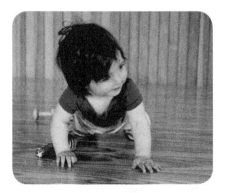 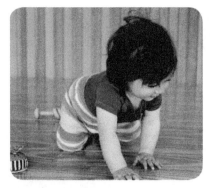

Bear-walks with hands and feet on the floor, behind up

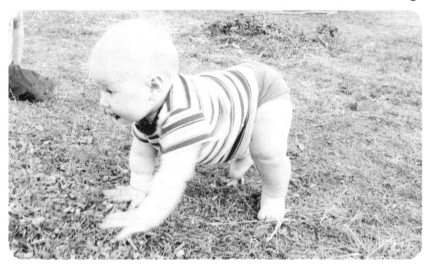

Hands-and-knees to side-sitting

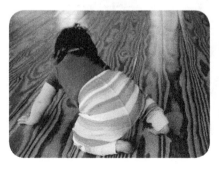 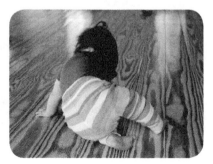

Sits back from crawling and plays in kneeling

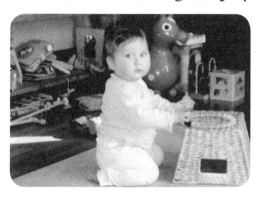

Walks on knees

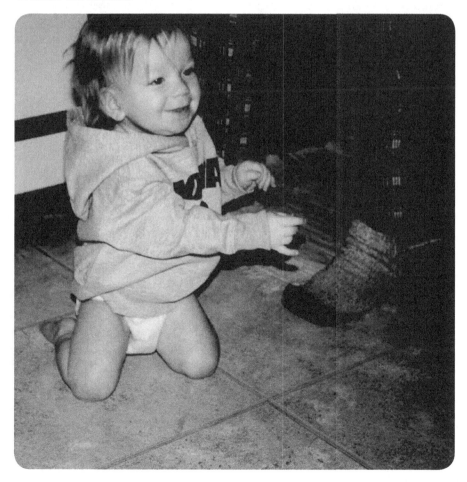

Pulls to standing, rolls over tops of feet (early standing)

Plants one foot, then pushes up to stand

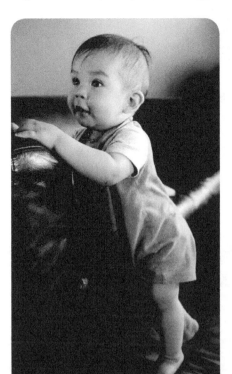

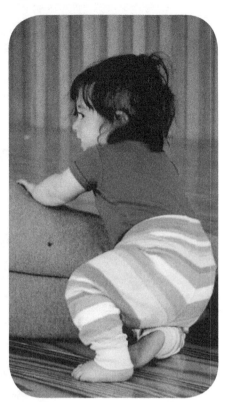

Drops down intentionally from standing to sitting

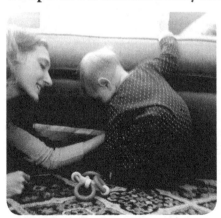

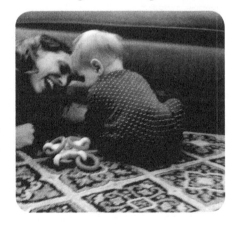

Stands holding onto something

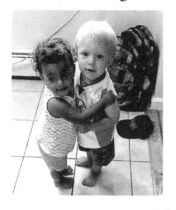

Squats down from standing

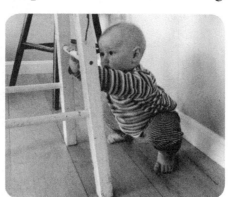

Side-steps while holding onto something stable

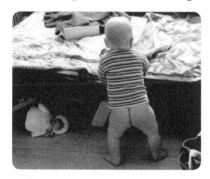 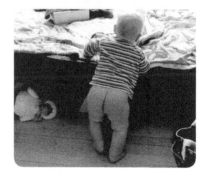

Steps forward independently

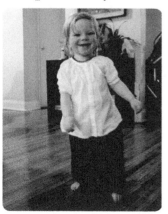

Toddles off - bye bye!

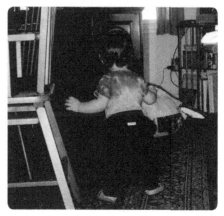

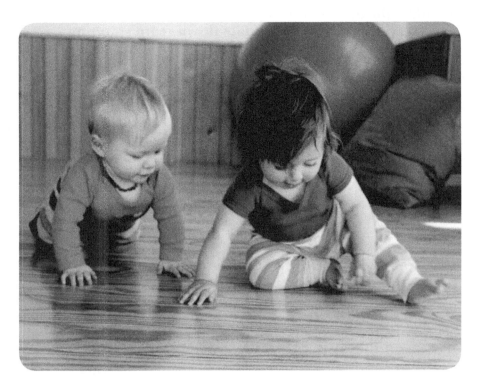

Friendship on the way.

Helping Baby Learn to Move Naturally *Leads to:*

- *many months of independent movement on the floor before standing.*

- *appropriate capacity for self-regulation.*

- *less startling, less crankiness, and easier communication.*

- *emotional and physical confidence.*

- *healthy core-strength, less falling in sitting and walking.*

- *more enjoyment in, and coordination of, fine and gross motor play.*

- *life-long strength and flexibility in body and mind.*

Foundational Early Months

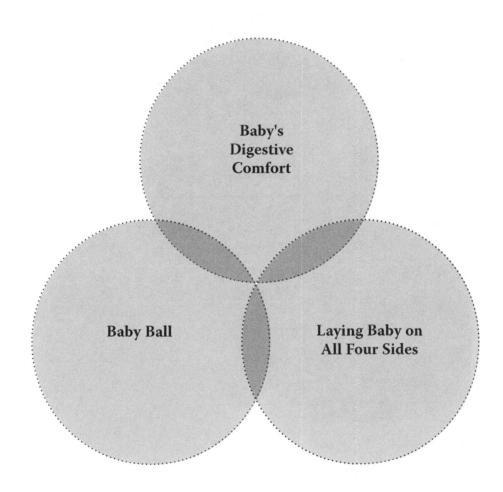

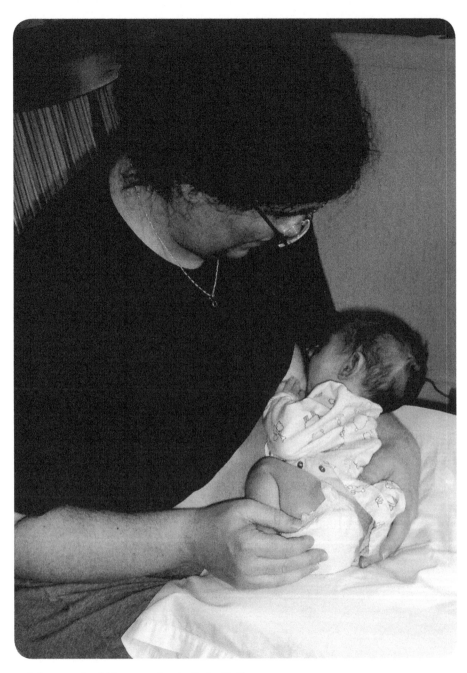

A four-week-old boy nursing in Baby Ball.

2. Baby Ball

Baby Ball is a core practice in Natural Movement Development and supports all the rest of the practices. Baby Ball provides *flexion* with *compression* for Baby, which are essential for healthy development. Muscles on the front of the body are called flexors. Curling the spine forward around the belly button is flexion. Muscles on the back of the body are called extensors. Arching is *extension*.

Flexion begins when Baby is growing in his mother's uterus. He is curved around his umbilical cord in a ball-like shape,

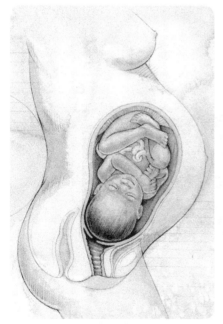

increasingly compressed from all sides as he grows. This is Baby's home base. His nervous system begins its growth here. After he's born and as he continues to grow, Baby benefits from returning regularly to this flexed and compressed position, which I call *Baby Ball*. This is a fundamental position for resting and recharging in infancy and throughout his life.

This drawing shows a fetus flexed and compressed in his eighth month in utero.

Repeat Flexion On the Way

Baby requires reinforcement in flexion positions
as he gains each new movement skill. Baby tends
to learn each movement through extension and
needs help to find and use flexion at every
stage of development; this is natural.

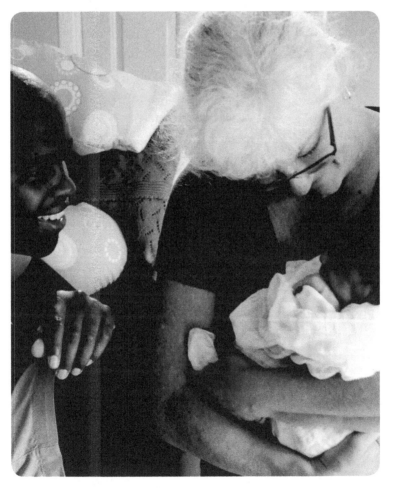

This father enjoys seeing his 2-week-old girl relax in Baby Ball.

Extension, Flexion, and Compression

Baby grows naturally when held often in his Baby Ball. Stress *in utero*, during birth, or in the earliest hours, whether mild or severe, intensifies his strength on the back of his body, making him strong in his *extensor** muscles after he is born. When Baby's extensor muscles ares stronger than his flexor muscles, he will have to work harder to find his way up from the floor, and from upset to comfort. Back strength and front strength are both natural and good. The difference is that extension is mostly learned automatically, while Baby needs help building flexion into each new movement skill. We can fertilize his development by lovingly adding flexion to comfort and play.

Providing Baby with flexion and compression calms him and supports full, natural reflex development. Part of why Baby arches easily is because any *startle*, small or large, causes extensor muscles on the back of the body to strengthen. Flexor muscles, on the other hand, are triggered by being held with compression. Teaching parents the necessity and practices of flexion that Baby needs is a large part of what this book offers.

There are many reasons why Babies become better at thrusting and arching in extension rather than at pulling in with flexion. Some of these are:

- Parents thinking arched-back baby is relaxed.
- Parents not knowing that Baby needs to be flexed.
- Cultural value that upright sooner is better. Early uprightness makes arching and thrusting stronger.

- Frequent propping from an early age makes certain reflexes, those that engage extensor muscles, overactive.
- A belief that Baby is smarter and cuter when he is upright. (Yet, he's just as cute when he's horizontal! This is where he learns to sit without you doing it for him.)

This book will help you better understand and provide flexion for your Baby. And, because each growth spurt increases extension, Baby will need help to learn and re-learn flexion. In fact, the more loose and relaxed Baby seems, the more he needs compression at each stage of motor-growth to help him develop balanced strength, coordination, and attention.

Balanced strength in flexing and extending allows Baby to achieve his primary independent movements more easily.

Babies born prematurely or under stress tend to startle more easily than those who come to full-term without enduring stress at birth. When babies receive life-saving care in the hospital, they spend most of the time on their backs. Flexion positions are helpful for alleviating the overactive *startle reflex* that is caused by exclusive back-lying. Baby Ball provides calming flexion which helps reflexes to develop naturally.

While flexion is natural, and *flexion to flexion** is natural, I've found most parents benefit from a better understanding of how to provide Baby with flexion in daily life. This understanding lets you help Baby return to his original feelings of contained comfort as he moves into his surroundings.

My work with infants ranges from those who are robust and born easily to those who were stressed in birth. Some of these children are more frail than average with special needs that are acute or long-term.

With all infants, I find the majority have stronger extensor muscles than flexor muscles. I observe that this extension contributes to, and indicates, the challenges that both well and special-needs babies both can experience.

These challenges include movement issues such as:
- Frequent startling.
- Frequent back-arching and leg-thrusting.
- Crying while on the tummy.
- Lying down, not rolling.
- Sitting, not moving.
- Moving by inch-worming on the back.
- Unusual or delayed uttering and speech.
- Standing, not having crawled.

Organic issues such as:
- Difficulty falling or staying asleep.
- Painful gas.
- Reflux.
- Colic.
- Asthma.

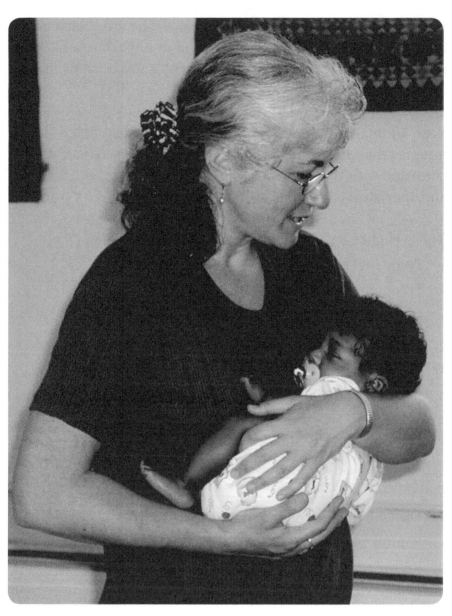

This five-week-old boy rests in Baby Ball with Lenore.

(P)ractice

Baby Ball

Baby Ball practice gives Baby flexion and compression. This is his physical and neurological "home base," part of his bond with you. It is similar to the firm containment he felt in the womb but is more flexible.

Hold Baby in a firm ball against your body. Have one of your arms behind his head and neck, the other arm under his thigh.

Bring his knees toward his belly until his back is in a C-shaped curve. Keep his head in line with his spine or bent just slightly forward, not with his neck bent back.

He may arch his back and thrust both his legs out, or just one leg or the other. This is fine. Let him fully extend arching his back.

Wait while he extends and maintain your arms around his knees as he moves. Arching is cyclical. It will be strong and then diminish. If you wait he will soften, even if only a little. During this softening, fold him into a ball with his knees toward his belly button. Hold him there gently and firmly with steady compression. Refrain from jiggling his legs in and out. Just hold them steadily until he is done.

Practice Baby Ball with Baby in your arms first then explore Baby Ball in nursing, on your shoulder, and in your lap. (Please see pg. 106 for more on crying while arching and then re-grouping to Baby Ball).

Flexion-to-Flexion

When Baby nuzzles into your body, you fold
your body and arms around Baby. I call this the
flexion-to-flexion reflex. The sound and sensation
of your heartbeat, so near in flexion-to-flexion,
deeply soothes Baby. The feeling of Baby's body
can also soothe the adult who flexes around him.

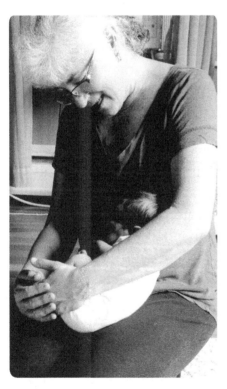 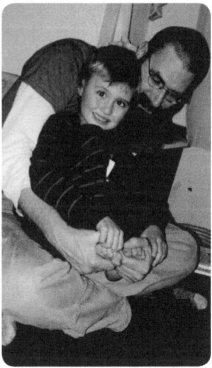

Parent as Flexion Teacher

Baby benefits from your help to return to a ball-shaped base all through his childhood. These are times of rest or comfort. With repetition, he relaxes into himself and into your body with his legs folded, his neck mildly flexed, and his spine in a *C-curve**. Use your body to give Baby containment with compression similar to what he felt in the womb. Flexion-to-flexion can be a natural, restorative, re-set time for you both.

Some of this relates to startle and recovery. Excitement is great periodically. Surprises can be fun, or upsetting. New things are great for Baby until he is done, and then he can get stressed. Providing a little recovery time after these stresses with gentle flexion is part of parenting naturally, although certainly some children may not enjoy it as often.

Being a flexion teacher helps make family life sustainable. It is a process, like gardening. Every time Baby grows in body and mind, you'll feel him increase in his back-arching and strong thrusting of his legs. Throughout his infancy and childhood, Baby needs you to 'fertilize' his body and mind with moments of restorative flexion. We don't aim to stop Baby's extension, we just keep trying to balance it with flexion.

> The moment the baby shifts from arch to you-can-mush-me-into-a-ball only comes through a willingness to wait for it. Somehow, this very simple action prepared me for other discomforts ahead. I could trust that the metaphoric arch wouldn't last forever. And you know what? It never does.
>
> *A Mother*

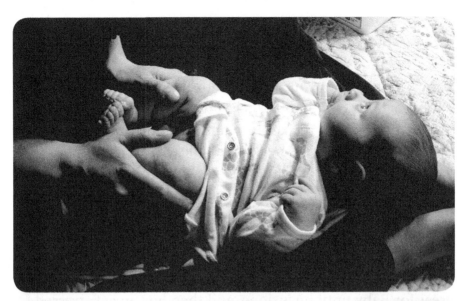

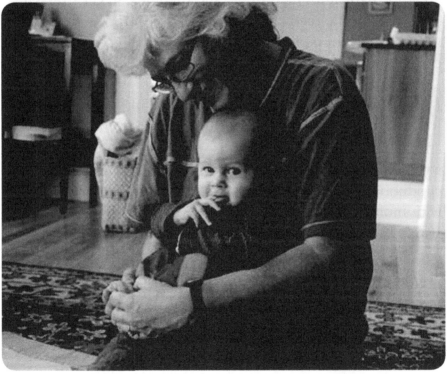

In these photos, Lenore helps a two-week-old and six-month-old respectively to flex both legs fully to the belly button. It feels good!

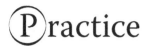ractice

Helping Baby Flex Both Legs

When Baby is young and is having a moment of quiet on his back, perhaps after a diaper-change, try gently and slowly to move both his knees toward his belly button.

If he is thrusting, wait and refrain from jiggling his legs. If you do jiggle, it usually causes him to thrust more. Your young baby may never have flexed so that his knees fully in to his belly and the inside surfaces of his legs touch, with the soles of his feet side by side.

Do this practice briefly and often. Don't make Baby stay in any position. Sometimes he will relax here when you hold his legs. Perhaps passing gas, defecating, or drifting off.

If Baby has strong thrusting, even if you practice flexing both legs when he is tiny, expect to continue to lovingly help Baby flex his legs and fold at the waist as he grows.

Baby Ball and Digestion

New parents are rarely told just how much of Baby's time will be spent digesting—and how uncomfortable his digestion might feel at times in the early months of his life.

In Baby's first weeks, he gets a lot of sensory input from his own digestive tube. Sometimes this input is startling or uncomfortable. Baby's earliest days may be stressful at times. Baby's digestive discomfort may feel alarming. It's hard to see Baby uncomfortable. But, because his digestive tube is immature at birth, his digestive sensations are not yet "white noise" for him as they are for adults.

Baby needs your help with his digestion. Getting settled in feeding, burping, and passing gas, all require your aid sometimes. When Baby's digestion bothers him, he has difficulty settling. All this takes time and care. Baby Ball is an essential practice for soothing and settling Baby. Baby's digestive comfort comes first and foremost in his development. First digestion then movement in space. Baby can catch up on movement, once his belly feels better.

>   We were amazed that our baby's chronic constipation was relieved when we learned to bend his thrusting legs—especially his right leg. I had no idea that was connected to digestion! Now, if he is uncomfortable when he is pooping I hold him on his left side and help him with his leg a little, and there is no problem—its amazing!
>
> *A Dad*

$\textcircled{P}$ractice

Baby Ball in Nursing

- Whether breast or bottle-feeding, give Baby time to settle after latching on.
- Next, help Baby into Baby Ball. Let him move his arms as he wishes. Gently, with your hand under his thighs, bend his knees towards his belly button.
- Then, position Baby so his neck is just slightly bent forward of his plumb line (straight up and down).
- Let him move his head onto the nipple instead of your inserting it while his neck is bent back.

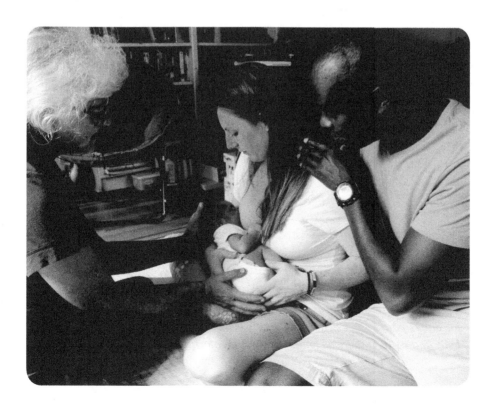

What's happening here?

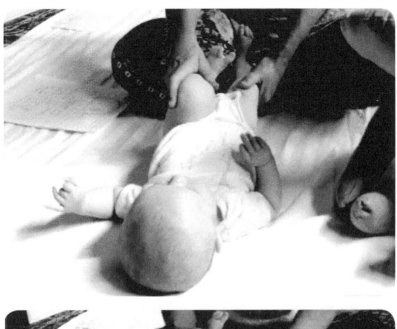

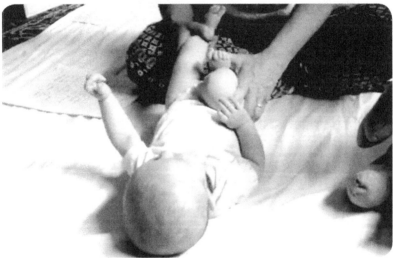

This two-month-old thrusts her right leg powerfully. Lenore waits for Baby's pause, then swiftly and gently brings her left knee to her belly and holds it there as long as Baby is comfortable.

(P)ractice

Flexing the Thrusting Leg

Sometimes when you are holding Baby in Baby Ball you will notice that he thrusts one leg or the other. His leg is long and strong. This is not a cause for concern. It is an indication to help him learn to flex his leg more easily.

• If Baby's leg is thrusting strongly, keep your hand on his foot and wait. At some point his thrust will soften, even if only a little and only briefly.

• With the softening, keeping your hand flat on the sole of his foot, bend his knee to his belly button and remain there.

• If he thrusts again, let him; keep your hand on his foot, ready to fold his leg again next time his thrust softens.

Babies have one leg they thrust more readily than the other. If he's constipated, it will likely be his right leg.

Practicing over time, Baby continues to thrust the same leg often. However, he will now also be able to bend that leg with more ease, and increase thrusting in his other leg. This is a valuable foundation for his belly crawling in the months ahead.

Continue to help Baby soften and fold into flexion. As well as flexing the more thrust-prone leg a little each day, continue to use Baby Ball as resource for comfort. This practice is especially relevant if Baby is constipated. Sometimes, moving Baby's right knee toward his belly helps his bowels to move.

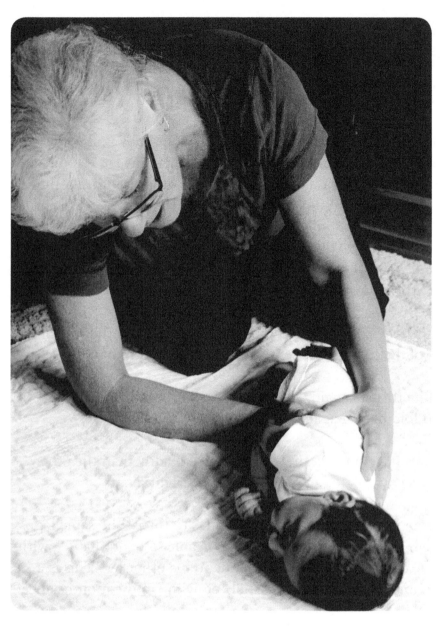

*Helping this month-old girl with her digestion, Lenore combines
laying Baby on her left side, bending her top leg, and gently massaging her
belly in and down.*

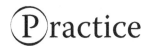ractice
Soothing Baby's Digestive Discomfort

Try These for Baby
- Hold Baby in Baby Ball. Offer him a chance to nurse, take his bottle, mouth your finger or his pacifier.
- Lay Baby on his left side. Gently bend his right knee toward his belly. He doesn't need to bend his leg all the way.
- Stroke Baby's torso slowly and firmly in a downward direction, with one hand on his front and the other on his back. This is especially helpful if Baby has reflux. Think 'in and down' as you stroke his body on his front and back.
- Give Baby a belly massage with organic oil. Massage slowly in an 'n' shape. Up from pelvis to ribs, across, and down from ribs to pelvis. Repeat. The part of Baby's intestine where it turns from across to down is often where he feels the most discomfort.
- Baby can have liquid probiotic in his bottle.

Try These for Nursing Mom
- Prepare Mom some fennel or spearmint tea in the evening.
- Introduce a probiotic. Take half the dose the first day. If the results are neutral or welcome, try the full dose. Nursing Baby can be given a probiotic from a dropper in addition to mother's milk.
- Remove one item from your diet such as dairy, wheat, onions and garlic, corn, or soy for five days. Next, add that food back to your diet for a day and note the results.

It is not necessary to do it all at once. This is an area to listen to your intuition as to what to try. Keep a record of what you tried, the date, and the results. If Baby's discomfort persists, seek outside assistance.

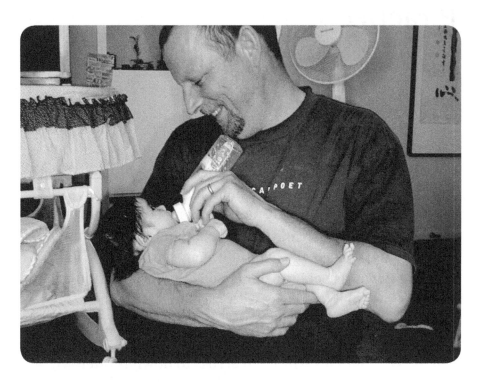

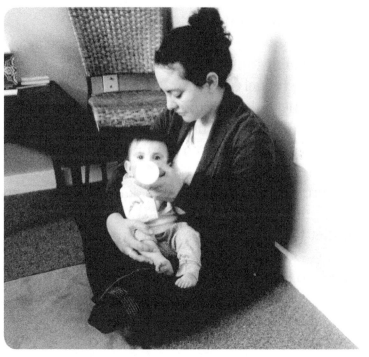

(P)ractice

Baby Ball with Nursing and Bottle-Feeding

If you are bottle-feeding, switch occasionally from holding Baby on one side of your body to the other, just as in breast-feeding.

If one side is more comfortable, try to use the other side at least some of the time during feeding and holding. Have pillows available to make holding Baby as comfortable for you as possible.

It helps Baby's digestive and nervous system if parents hold Baby in a soft Baby Ball position while bottle-feeding. Hold Baby tilted slightly back or on his side, rather than flat on his back. Support his head in slight flexion with one arm, put your other arm under his thighs bringing his knees toward his belly button. Over time help Baby learn to touch and hold his bottle while you flex him during bottle-feeding.

Support Your Body

Whether breast- or bottle-feeding, sit comfortably in a chair or against a support. Place a pillow under your arm or use whatever you need to decrease strain on your body.

Ⓟractice

Please Pass the Baby Ball

If you are holding Baby in his ball shape, and it's time to pass him to another grown-up, keep him in this shape as you pass him so you won't need to hang him by his armpits. As you do this, think "knees and nose to navel." Holding Baby's ball shape when you pass him avoids startling him which helps him to remain comfortable through the transition from one person to the other.

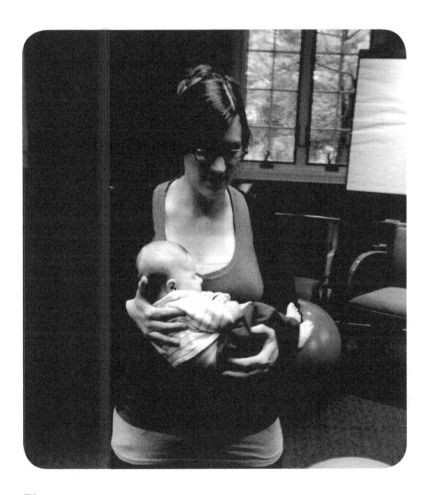

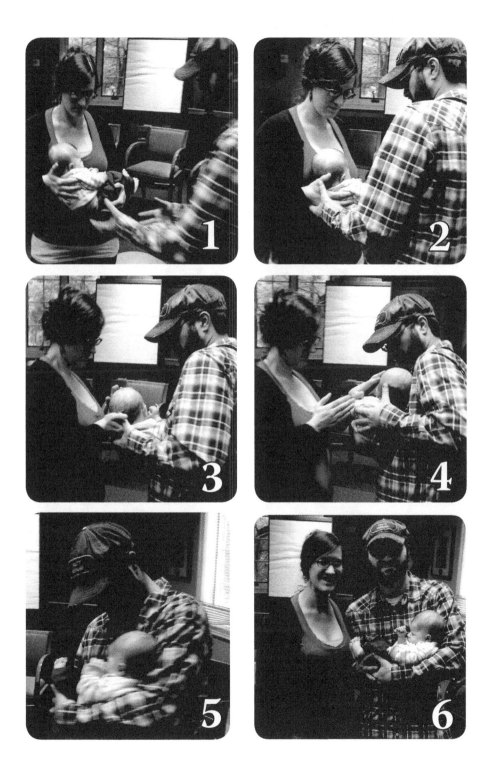

Regroup to Baby Ball
after Startle and Stress

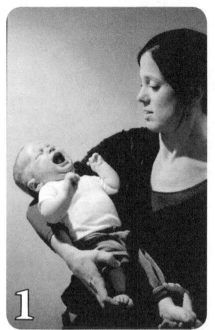

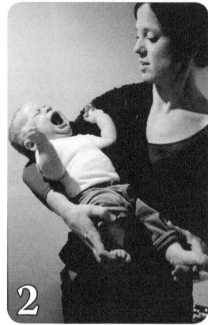

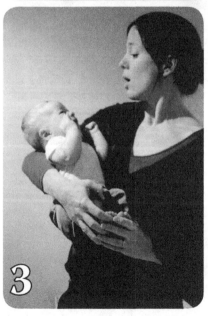

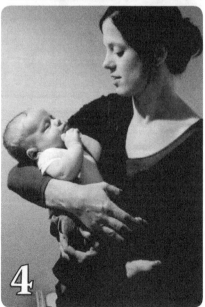

Try It Yourself

After stress, you might feel tension in your body.

Try taking a moment to unwind by stretching your arms up and out, while letting your back arch slightly. Say "blah: or "bleh" loudly to describe your upset. When done, let your arms down slowly, bring your hands in to rest comfortably on your chest. Mildly and gently flex your body so that your head is slightly forward, and rest here to give yourself some calming breaths or calming thoughts.

A similar thing happens when someone cares about us, and wants to listen to how we are. If you have had a hard time, I hope someone will listen kindly to you, without giving advice. When you get your story out, you might like a hug after (not always, you get to say). A hug is everyday flexion medicine.

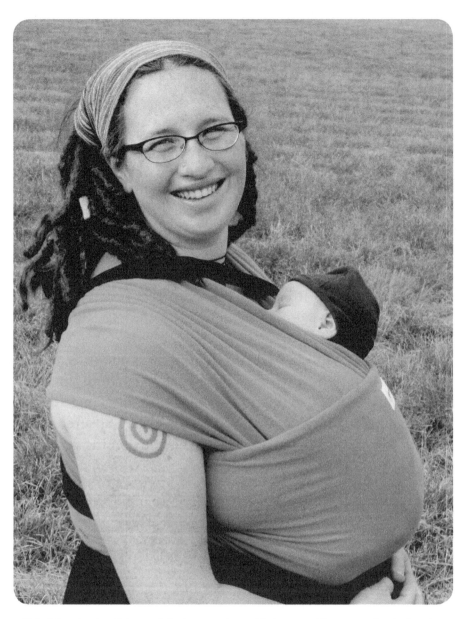

This Mom is practicing safe baby-wearing with her son. She wears her baby at "kissing distance" and can see her baby's face. Baby's neck is not too bent so his airways are clear.

Carriers that Support Baby Ball

Slings are a great way to keep Baby in his flexed Baby Ball position, particularly in his early months. When possible, choose carriers that hold Baby fully under his bottom.

If the sling is comfortable for you, it's a great way to keep Baby near you when he's resting or sleeping, and have your hands free. Men and women enjoy a variety of carriers. Wearing Baby can be especially nice for the non-nursing parent. Try on more than one brand and size, as each parent might need his or her own. A good fit is important.

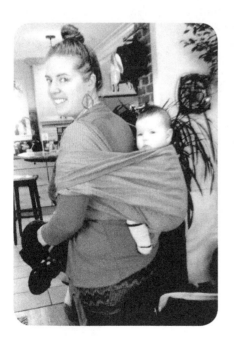 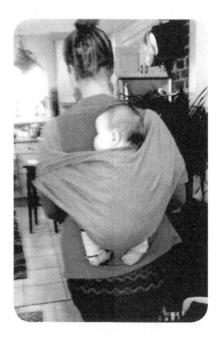

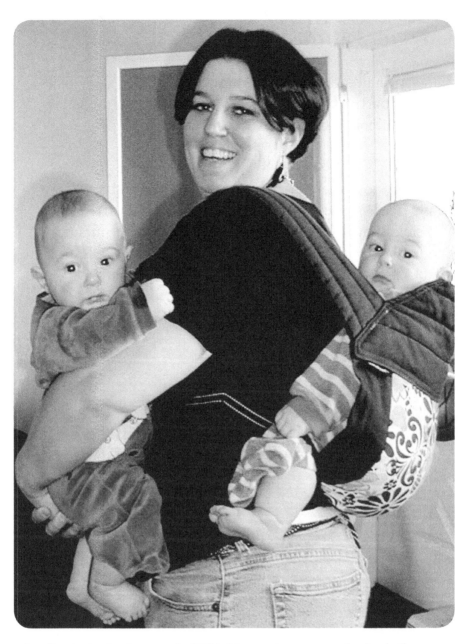

Aren't parents of twins amazing? This Mom puts one son on her back, then lifts her other son to her front. Off they go!

(P)ractice

Flexion Health with Wide-Leg Carriers

Parents ask if Baby's legs are spread open too widely in some carriers. The most important thing is to find a carrier that works for Baby and you. If it is one which spreads his legs wide, then take a moment to care for his hips after you take him out of the carrier.

• Put him down to lie, sit, or kneel where he is comfortable.

• Then, place your hands on his hips without doing anything. Just have your hands there while you connect, perhaps exchange eye-contact or a kiss.

• Next, place your hands on either side of his hips over the bone and press gently from both sides inward toward his middle.

Giving Baby this hands-on compression helps to alleviate the wide feeling in his hip joints after being in the carrier. It's a simple way to reduce your worry and it's a short feel-good squish that you and Baby have as a routine after getting out of the carrier.

It is best to avoid carriers that dangle Baby by his crotch with no support under his bottom.

Natural Alternatives to Moving Baby by His Armpits

It's so easy to pick Baby up by his armpits, because he is moved passively from one place to another. You may not have been told that there are other ways to pick Baby up. Holding Baby by his armpits is necessary at times. Yet, often, alternatives can be used, such as:

• maintaining Baby in his ball shape as you move him.

• leaning Baby to his side, slide one hand under his hip and the other under his neck, and lift him up at an angle.

• putting one hand behind his neck, slide one hand under his bottom, and lift him from your bottom hand.

• sliding your forearm under his front when he is on his belly and lift him this way.

Let Family and Friends Do It Their Way

There is not a right or wrong way to hold Baby. People have their own way of holding Baby and their own reasons why they do it that way. Try not to worry or to criticize their methods. The love and the relationship is always most important!

If someone asks, show them an alternative way to hold Baby. Keep it simple and let Baby's attention lead.

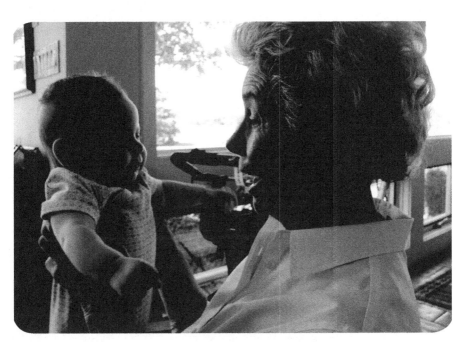

The granddaughter and grandmother admiration society is in session.

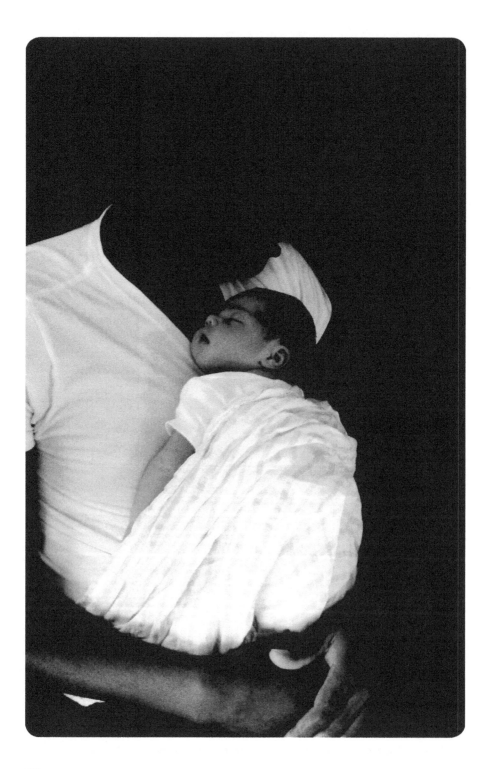

On the Way to Walking

Taking Care Along the Way

Baby brings indescribable love and joy to your life. Sometimes he brings exhaustion, or feelings of overwhelm.

Not every parent is exhausted, but most are tired for some part of the first year of Baby's life. Even if you are one of the lucky few who are getting enough sleep, you are still absorbing this tremendous change in your life and your lifestyle. Who knew you could spend so many hours feeding Baby, doing laundry, and then feeding Baby and doing laundry?

When you are overtired, you might think that you are not doing enough or not doing it "right." Unfortunately this is a common feeling, yet is not true. I think what might be true is that you are tired because you are parenting, and tiredness can shed a difficult light on your day.

For this small moment, take a deep breath and short rest.

Sometimes couples separate for naps, or even for night sleeping, for a period. If sleeping separately to tend to Baby, dates for a snuggle are greatly appreciated.

What are they doing?

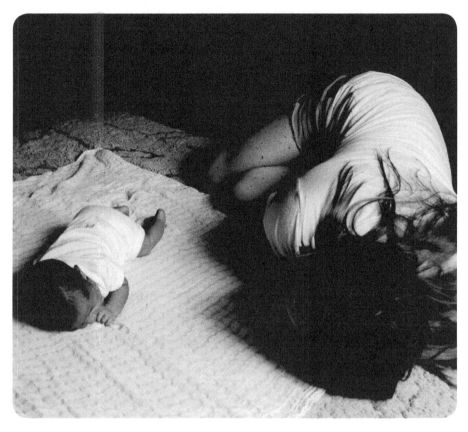

Mom is resting on her side in flexion keeping sweet company with her baby.

Try It Yourself

Restful Flexion

To understand restful flexion, it's ideal to experience it. Make a time to lie on your side in a ball. Let your arms and legs bend comfortably toward your belly button. Use a small pillow so your neck is relaxed. When you first lie down, just notice your position. Slowly, explore bringing your knees just a little closer to your belly, and letting your neck bend just a little more forward so your nose points toward your feet.

If you feel like stretching out your whole body into a big long arch, then coming back to flexion, it will probably feel even more comfortable than before you stretched.

You may prefer one leg tucked over the other in a particular way, or you may usually keep one hand closer to your face than the other. Note your familiar choices in flexion.

This is a moment of ease for you. I know that reading this book might feel overwhelming. The information might at first make life with Baby feel more complicated. I have seen that once a parent goes through the learning curve, things feel easier. The practices become a natural part of parenting. Knowing this, have a little break in restful flexion.

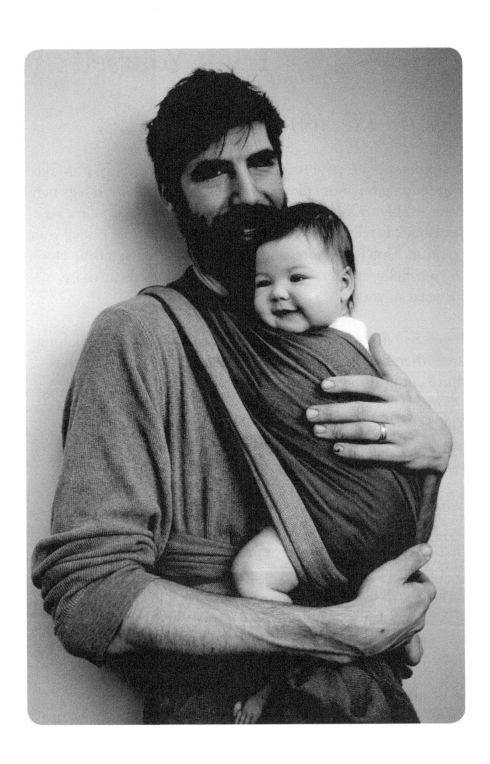

Baby Ball *Leads to:*

- *bonding between Baby and you.*
- *improved digestion for Baby, including better resolution of painful gas.*
- *comfortable InnerTime for Baby.*
- *Baby's ability to self-regulate.*
- *more confidence for you when soothing Baby.*
- *independent side-lying.*
- *more comfort and fun in TummyTime.*

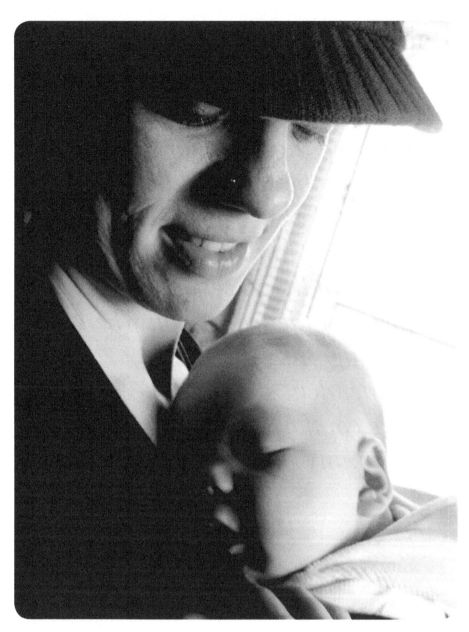

A Mom supports her two-week-old's InnerTime.

3. Protect Baby's Early InnerTime

The first three months stand alone as a precious period in Baby's life. He is bonding with you and the world. He is learning to see, to move his head on his neck, to digest and to sleep comfortably.

In this first chapter of his life, he will likely be alert for brief periods. His alert time is a great time to play with him and enjoy eye contact. However, most of the time his attention will be focused inwardly. It's important to let him have this InnerTime. He wants to be held by you, to feel your body, and hear your familiar heartbeat. You do not have to always stimulate him or relate to him with eye contact. Meeting Baby where his attention is simplifies your life and will help support Baby's development.

As an adult, you are far more accustomed to face-to-face eye contact than Baby. When Baby is resting on your body, he is relating to you through his whole being. He feels your warmth, he hears your heartbeat and he is moved by your breathing. Your protection of Baby's early InnerTime is a valuable investment in his ability to rest, digest, and bond. A foundation he builds on for the rest of his life.

Slowly, Baby's focus will expand. He will be perceiving and moving toward more and more of the outside world. When you let Baby lead InnerTime, you allow him to show you his own self-regulation. Through this skill, he teaches you what he needs and when.

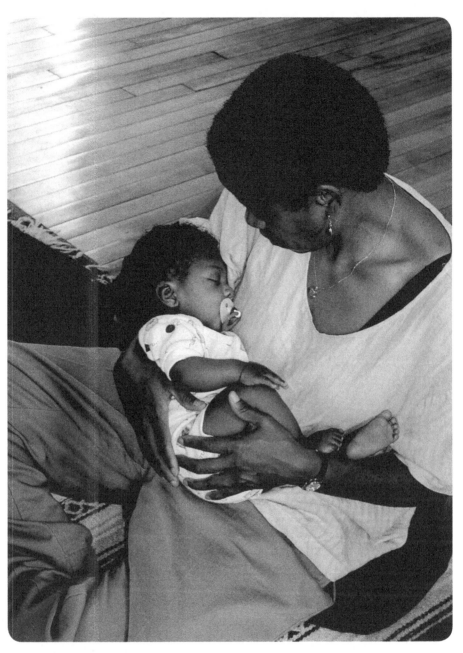

Mom helps her five-week-old rest in flexion as she flexes around him.

Feeling Blue

InnerTime is important for parents too. Some parents, whether biological or not, might be surprised to find themselves feeling a bit blue for a few days after Baby arrives. This happens often and is natural, due primarily to hormone changes. If your blue feeling persists for more than a few days, you may have postpartum depression. There is help for you. Start with: www.motherwoman.org

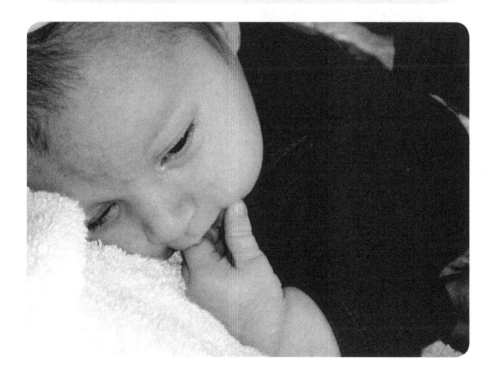

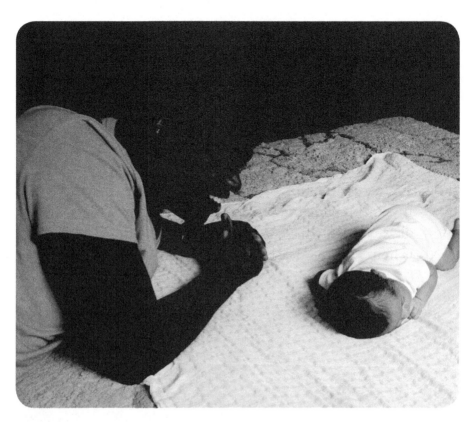

Dad with his new daughter.

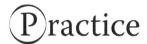ractice

Letting Baby Turn Away

Allow Baby to turn away and rest when he chooses to.

Some of your visitors, or folks you encounter when you are out with Baby, express a lot of excited delight to see your new baby. What's not to delight?

Yet for you, and for Baby especially, it may be too much stimulation. If it is, simply say he needs to take his nap now, or find some other gentle way of protecting your baby.

Babies don't adhere to politeness. Try not to ask them to talk to the lady, or smile at Mrs. So-and-So. Let him look when he wants to, and turn away when he wants, especially in his first few months.

Of course, some babies are more social than others. Yet all will get tired, need to rest, and be startled by a face they weren't expecting, or have not seen, and a voice they do not know.

Baby may look with great curiosity at people, particularly new people. However, right now Baby is primarily on his foundational program, in which he eats, digests, sleeps, and bonds with his immediate people.

❝❝ Take time to explore picking up and holding your baby to increase your ease and confidence. Enjoy the moment; you are discovering a new relationship.

When you are ready to pick your baby up, give him your full attention, look at him, bring your body towards his, and wait for his eyes to meet yours. This encourages him to experience being lifted as a combined effort. Now, slide one hand under his neck and head, and your other hand under his behind. This supports the two heaviest parts of his body and reduces pressure on his joints. If you choose, you can gently turn Baby on his side before you lift him.

As you bring your body close to baby, curl his body towards you with his arms and limbs folded in, and cradle him against your chest. Bringing his weight to your center of gravity minimizes stress on your back. Keep your thumbs close to your fingers, and your hands in a straight line with your wrists when you lift baby, to protect the health of your wrists and shoulders.

As you lift baby, lean back, so that your body rather than your arms moves his weight. Arrange baby so that you support his head and gather all of his limbs. Take a moment to sense your own body, if there is tension in your arms, neck, or hands, breathe and allow yourself to relax. Your relaxation helps baby. ❟❟

Jamrog, S., (*Picking Up and Holding Your Baby: section from unpublished manuscript*).

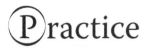ractice

Letting Baby Set the Rhythm

As much as you can, let Baby set the rhythm of your days and nights during your first months together. This does not spoil Baby; rather it helps him adjust to his new life.

Follow his lead as he transitions from awake to asleep, hungry to full, curious to quiet, and everything in between. Some days he nurses for hours; others, he sleeps more. Some nights he might cry long and hard, and other nights are mostly peaceful.

These different days don't occur in a predictable fashion. Routines arise, fall away, and new ones form as baby keeps changing. Keeping daily life simple gives you room to roll with the unpredictable and ever-changing young baby.

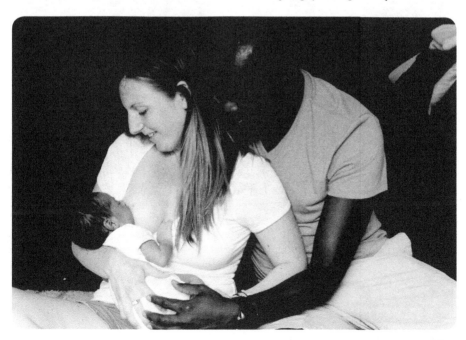

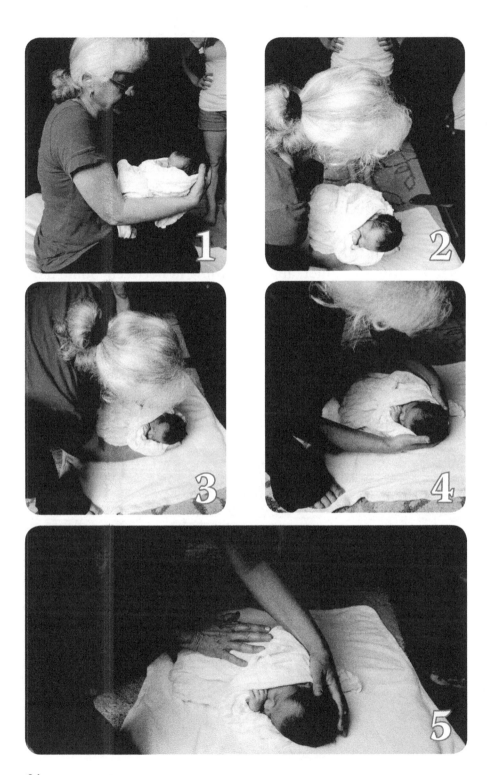

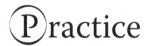

Practice

Transferring Your Sleeping Baby

The hope is to transfer Baby without triggering his startle reflex. As you move Baby from a car-seat, place one hand behind his head and neck, the other under his thighs with his legs to his belly. Keep him in this ball shape as you pick him up, with his head and knees folded in toward his belly button. If you allow his head to drop back or his legs to hang down while lifting him, he is more likely to startle. This is a natural response, and many babies will wake up when this happens.

It may take practice to lift him without waking him. Some babies just won't be able to stay asleep when you do this; others will.

Whenever possible, have a sleeping basket nearby or a flat, clean surface ready. Place him on his side to help him remain slightly flexed. From there you can roll him slowly to his back or let him remain on his side with a towel behind him.

While it's beneficial not to overuse the portable car-seat, there are exceptions. There may be times when the car-seat is what works for you and Baby. If Baby often sleeps in the car-seat, be sure to practice holding his hips in flexion on a daily basis.

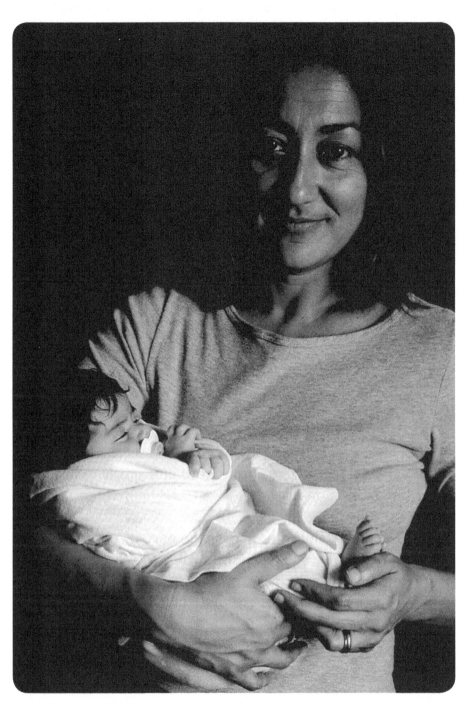

One-week-old girl swaddled comfortably in the Baby Ball with her pacifier, relaxing in flexion-to-flexion with Mom.

Pacifiers

Pacifiers are a personal choice for each family.
They can be helpful at times.

Pacifiers can fulfill the need of Baby's strong *sucking reflex**.
In this case, the pacifier is useful for Baby when he is not
hungry, but he needs to suck to soothe, especially if he has
painful gas.

If mother's nipples are irritated, the pacifier can provide
essential time for her to heal. In instances where Baby has a
disorganized or weak sucking reflex, the pacifier can help
strengthen the reflex and give Baby better nourishment.

Other stressors may also indicate a place for a pacifier in
Baby's life. Pacifiers are most indicated when there is
digestive discomfort. If Baby has reflux, the pacifier can be
an important tool for self-soothing. It helps Baby's esophagus
move the acid back down to the stomach.

If you are using a pacifier with your baby, keep several handy.
Try attaching them by a clip in several locations such as the
changing table, kitchen, and car. Try more than one size and
type, so you can see which he likes best. Offer it to Baby, but
do not persist if he pushes it away. Baby will latch on right
away if he needs to suckle to calm his system. If he needs to
cry, he will reject the pacifier. It's easy to see the difference
when you are looking for it.

Baby Ball can reduce the need for a pacifier over time.
But a pacifier sometimes helps Baby to relax into Baby Ball.

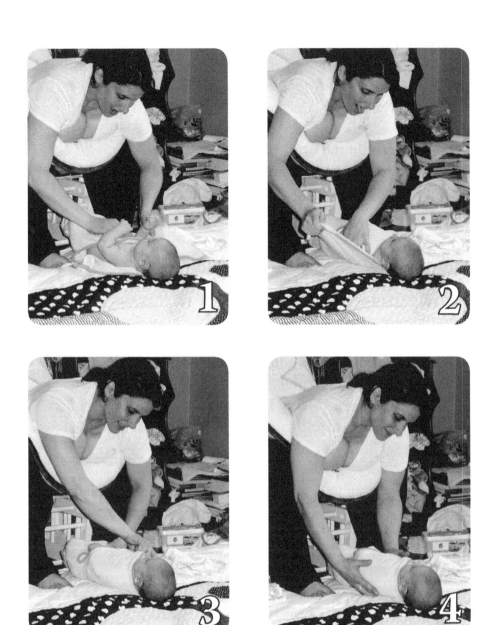

This Mom uses a swaddle-sack with velcro tabs to quickly wrap and settle her boy.

Swaddling

Swaddling is such a valuable daily resource for Baby and you. Some families have routine times of day that Baby is swaddled. Others swaddle Baby when he is tired and ready for sleep. Most newborns need lots of swaddle-time to settle.

Try swaddling Baby often in the first few months. Wrap him firmly in a soft cloth with his knees bent. This helps him maintain his ball position, which supports him to rest and digest.

If Baby doesn't seem to like swaddling, continue to introduce the option every other day. Sometimes a baby who cried during initial swaddling may grow to tolerate and be comforted by it.

Swaddle sacks are available with Velcro or snap closure. Some families swear by these.

For parents who choose to wear Baby during the earliest weeks, there is little chance to put baby down to swaddle him. No worries, he is getting what he needs while you wear him: firm compression similar to swaddling, wrapped against you.

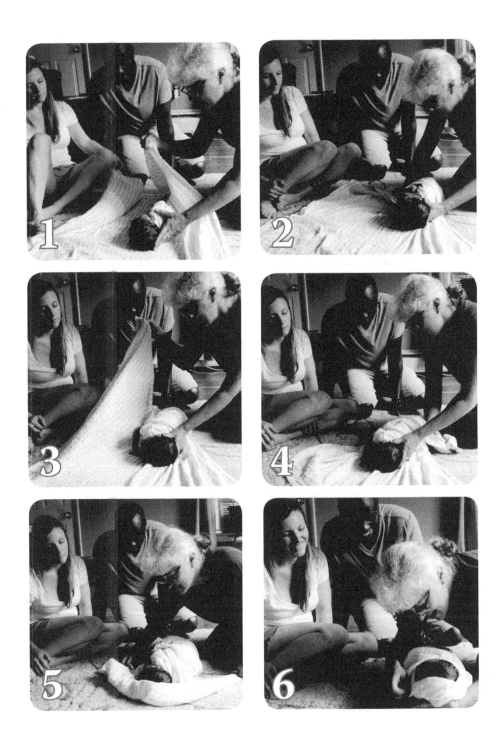

Ⓟractice

Swaddling Day-To-Day

Choose a swaddle fabric and practice wrapping a rolled towel. Follow the pictures here, or watch a video for your particular swaddle product.

Times when Baby appreciates being swaddled:

- after nursing and burping.
- after a short play time on his back with active random movements.
- after upset or startle.
- after diaper change.
- after a bath.
- before sleep.

Try placing Baby on his side with a rolled up towel behind him to keep him from rolling back.

Every Swaddle is Different

Your baby will be strong at thrusting his legs. At times he won't have any choice but to thrust, due to his reflexes. Swaddling gives Baby needed rest from thrusting by providing flexion and compression.

Every parent has their own comfort level with swaddling. For some it's so easy, and for others it feels awkward. Find your own way of folding the fabric or purchase a pre-made swaddle sack.

If you have been swaddling Baby regularly, there comes a point when you wonder if it is time to discontinue this practice. This often occurs when Baby's sleep schedule changes and when Baby has been playing contentedly in TummyTime. It is different for each child as to how long swaddling is needed. It is usually several months, but it can be shorter, and some might enjoy blankets and swaddling into childhood.

If you are curious about stopping swaddling, try slow reduction in frequency. Perhaps switch from twice a day to once, or only for napping or night time. You might try to swaddle Baby's lower body, leaving his arms free, for a few weeks. Either way, avoid a sudden stop if possible.

A Review of Supports for InnerTime

All of the preceding practices—and the ones you will devise on your own—work together throughout the day and over the weeks to support Baby's InnerTime in the earliest months. These include:

• Flexion to flexion.

• Resting with Baby.

• Swaddling.

• Awareness and care when Baby startles.

• Paying empathic attention to Baby when he cries.

• Letting Baby set the rhythm.

• Putting Baby's digestive comfort first. Soothing digestion with your "in and down" touch.

• Pacifier if helpful.

• Letting Baby turn away.

• Turning off screens, turning down lights.

• Playing gentle music.

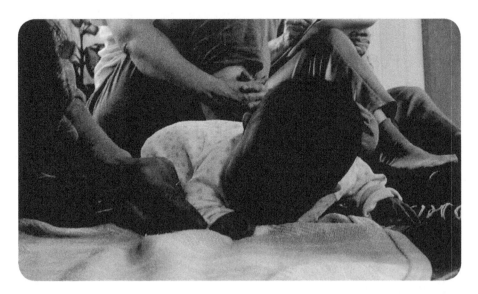

Mother helps Baby by keeping her company and touching her gently while Baby learns to turn her head while on her tummy.

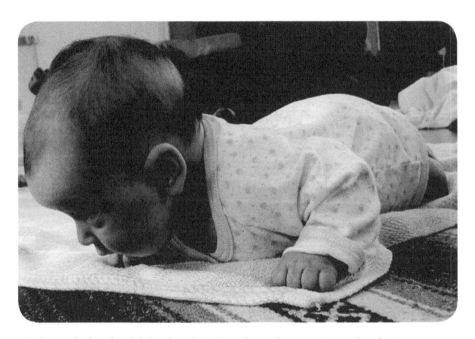

Baby works hard to lift her head. In this photo she experiences her first success at looking straight ahead while in TummyTime.

Alert Moments Early On

After a few months of mostly InnerTime, Baby's attention is outward more often. He lifts and turns his head with more ease, his face looks a bit more defined, and his gaze is more intentional. In these alert moments there is nothing you have to do, especially you don't have to be entertaining. Be present, engage with Baby, and enjoy.

Most often during TummyTime, Baby might rest quietly or focus on his own hand or on something nearby. Then, there are moments when he works to lift his head and look around. He will turn his head to the other side if he can, and let it down heavily after he has turned. What a big job!

Left and Right Build The Middle

Babies are initially able to hold their heads to the left or right. By doing so, they build the strength to hold their heads in the middle. It is a common assumption that the middle is an easier position than left or right. However, Baby is born with a tendency to be turned in one direction, then learns to turn in the other direction, and, from this moving back and forth, he builds strength to stay in the middle. Building the middle is a process Baby repeats at each stage, such as side-stepping and climbing.

A Bit On Crying

Baby cries to communicate his hunger, discomfort, and his need for your company. You respond with your reassuring attention, offering your breast or a bottle, perhaps checking his diaper.

Other times, Baby cries in order to release stress when he's tired, sad, or afraid. Care for him with this crying by staying with him, with your loving attention, holding him and letting him cry until he's finished. If he has a strong startle reaction to something, often he will cry until his startle is finished.

Often, parents learn to distinguish the cries for hunger or tiredness from the need to cry to release stress. Your focused listening is what he needs most to be able to release and recover.

Being a loving, gentle parent doesn't exclude that Baby might just need to cry at times. Do your best to let him cry until he's done, holding him calmly. Moving and cooing gently might help both of you.

Baby's discharging may feel scary to you sometimes. He can be surprisingly loud and cry at length with his whole body tense. This is natural, and you'll notice that usually he's peaceful afterward.

Sometimes Baby is 'telling his story' about his experiences, the fun, interesting ones and the uncomfortable, startling ones too. Crying helps Baby 'wipe his blackboard clean,' he processes the experiences of his day, so he can then shift into InnerTime, or feel refreshed for play.

Acknowledge and empathize with whatever Baby may be feeling. Gently attend to him while he expresses his feelings. You don't have to fix anything.

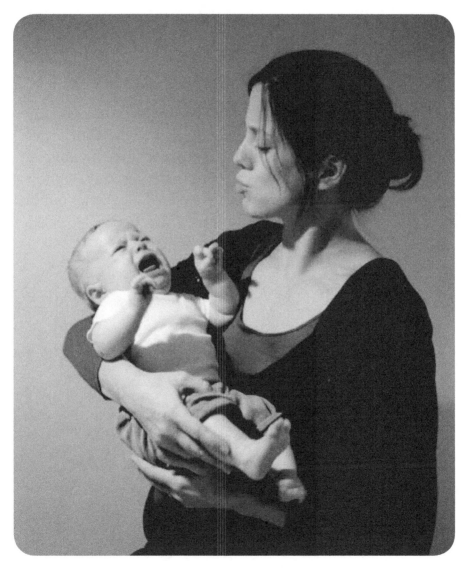

Three-month-old arching and crying while Mom listens empathically.

Baby's feelings, just like yours, don't necessarily make sense. He is never manipulating you or exaggerating or being dramatic. He is trying to heal himself in the most natural way possible, by discharging with your calm attention.

Hold Baby in your loving arms when he cries; make it your practice to stay as calm as you can. Baby uses your attention to take care of himself. His discharge is not the feelings, it is the healing.

When Baby cries you might have feelings of your own, maybe fear that you are not good enough, or frustration that you can't solve the crying. This is a clue that it might be helpful for you to find a time to share your own feelings with an empathic listener, ideally when Baby is asleep. After you receive some kind attention, it will be easier for you when Baby cries out his stress. You will both feel better after.

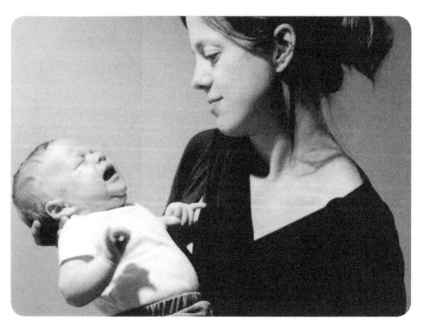

Mom calmly lets Baby cry.

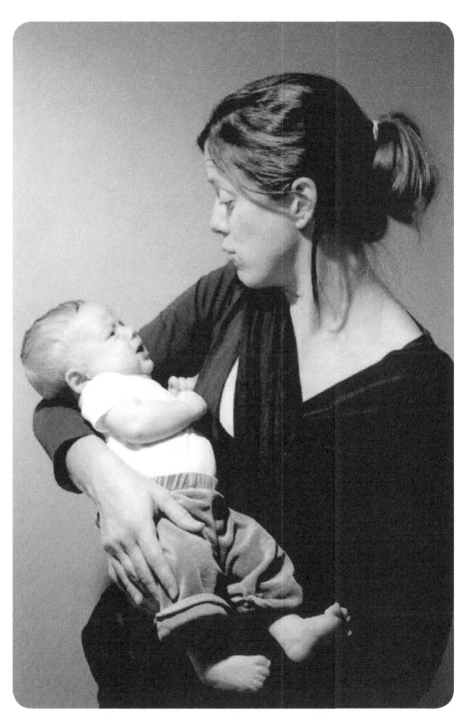

Mom shows Baby how much she cares with loving attention.

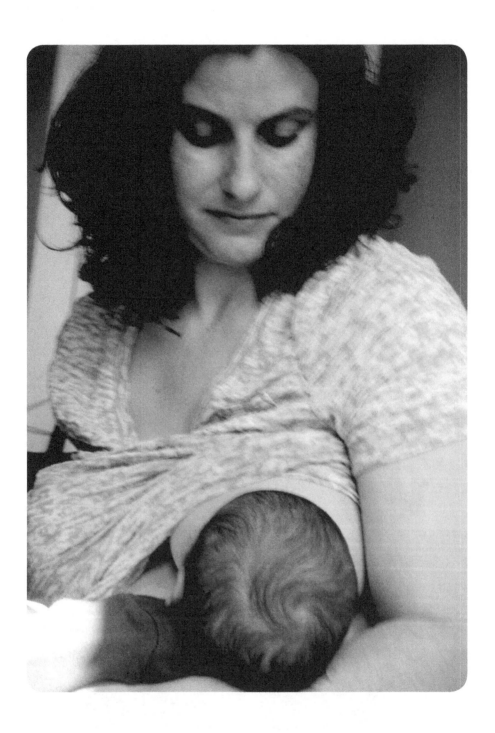

Protecting Early InnerTime
Leads to:

- *more rest and comfort for both of you.*
- *an easier time making Baby Ball part of everyday life.*
- *better ability to understand Baby's rest signals.*
- *Baby's natural recovery from stimulation.*
- *Baby's ability to sleep more readily.*
- *less strong arching and thrusting.*
- *resting, moving, and playing on all four sides.*

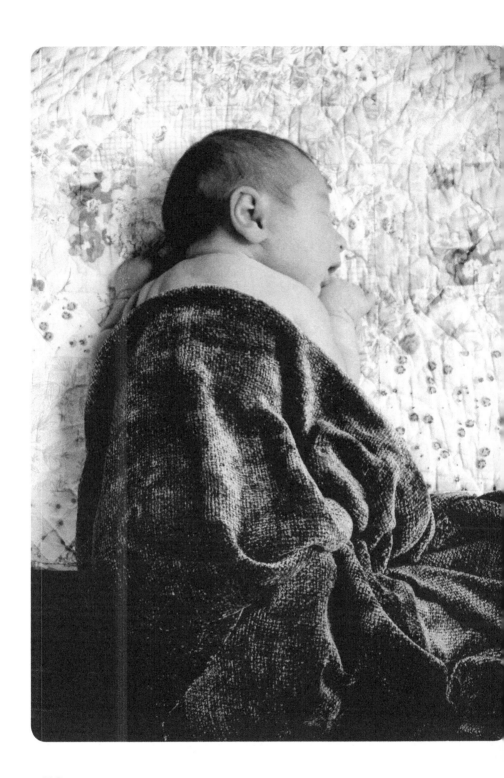

On the Way to Walking

4. All Four Sides and the Familiar Side

Placing Baby on all four of her sides is one of the most basic and helpful things you can do for her reflex development. Lying on both her left and right side, she receives appropriate stimulation from gravity to her whole brain and body.

This stimulation is an essential part of Baby's development. Baby finds interesting things lying on each side. The combination of experience on all her sides opens the skills that help Baby with what comes in the months ahead, such as learning to roll, belly-crawl and sit.

Everyone has a more familiar and a less familiar side. Often parents notice that Baby turns her head to one side more than the other or prefers to lie on one side.

Sidedness is not a cause for alarm. It is not something that needs to be fixed. Because Baby was tucked more to one side than the other *in utero*, it is natural for him to be asymmetrical. In Natural Movement Development, parents consciously engage Baby's reflexes on both of her body halves.

Some Babies remain strongly sided, and others become more bilaterally flexible. My goal isn't perfect symmetry for Baby. It is for you to understand how to provide reflex opportunities for Baby to both sides.

Lying on Her Back

Baby can do a lot of things on her back. She's going to be spending a lot of time here, looking around, resting, bringing her hands to her mouth and touching her hands together. She can vocalize, turn her head, learn to swipe at, and then hold on to things. She enjoys easy eye contact with you here, and lots of talking, singing, kissing, and playing.

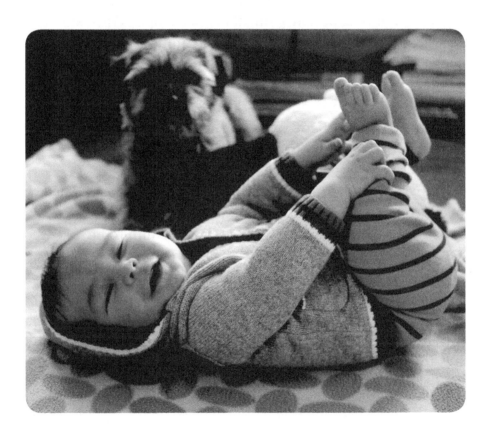

Lying on Her Left Side

Help Baby learn to lie on both sides by placing her there from the beginning. This is a natural position for Baby, one she needs you to provide for her. At first, put your hand on her pelvis and help her roll toward her side from her back. Soon, she'll do this herself. Lie on all four of your own sides in the TummyTime space, and help baby do the same.

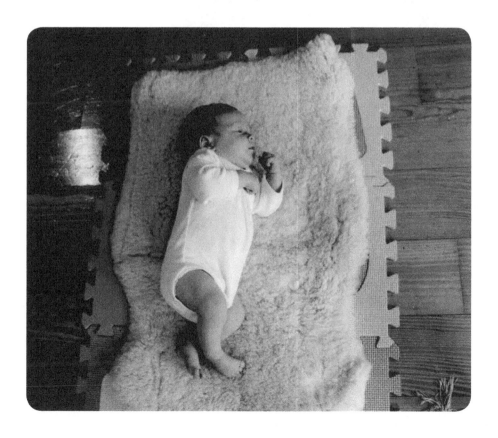

Lying on Her Right Side

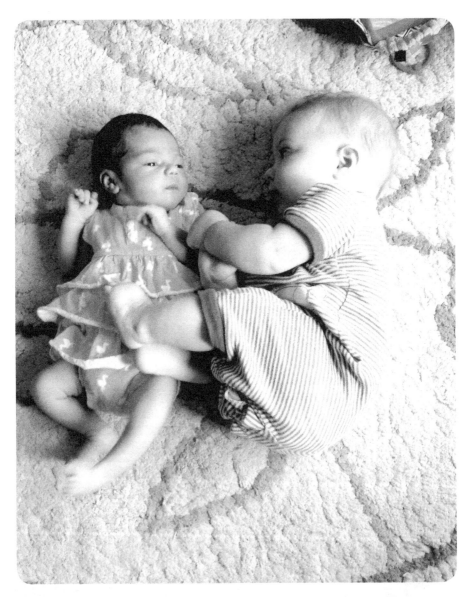

Babies love to visit. Here, the bigger baby has rolled towards the smaller one because he can.

Lying on Her Tummy

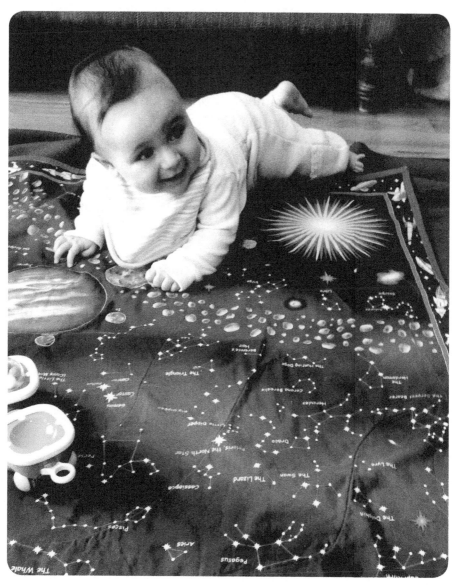

TummyTime is out of this world!

Random Movements

Random movements is the name of a reflex. When you lay Baby on her back without swaddling, you may see her move her arms and legs about actively. Sometimes she looks like she is "swimming" or "exercising." She is actually responding to the pull of gravity from her *low brain*, something she does automatically. That's what makes it a reflex.

While it is nice for her to have some clothing-free and diaper-free time to let her limbs move freely, she can easily tire from this and begin to cry, letting you know she wants a break from this reflex.

Random movements are natural and they are also tiring. After a diaper change, let Baby do her random movements on her back for a short time and then roll her to her left, her right, or her tummy, or swaddle her and hold her. (See pg. 105 for more on swaddling.)

Try It Yourself

Make a nice place for yourself on the floor. Lie down on your back and rest for a moment. Gently, when you are ready, let your arms and legs begin to lift and move as though they are floating in water. Your head and neck might respond with movement also. It may feel slow and thick or fluid and active. Either way, let yourself move until your breath softens. Feel your muscles lifting your limbs away from and back down towards gravity. Move without thinking; enjoy the freedom of your limbs. When you are finished, rest on your back again.

Roll to your side and use your arms to push up to sitting.

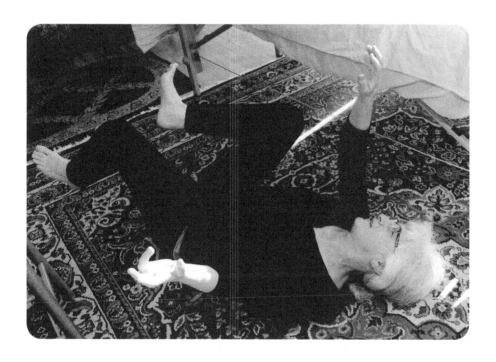

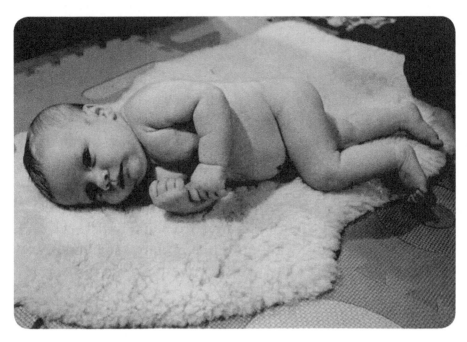

*This 3-month-old is having a sensory rich time with her diaper off.
She is learning to keep her balance in side-lying. Side-lying prepares her for
belly crawling later. This position helps to engage the reflexes of the big toe,
which she will use to push when she is ready to belly-crawl.*

Diaper-Free on All Four Sides

Whether your baby wears disposable or washable diapers, she will appreciate some time without one on. Place a stack of towels and a box of wipes at your TummyTime place and let Baby spend a few minutes a day feeling her body moving without her diaper. A large, washable, waterproof bed pad can be used underneath the blanket surface. Sometimes an absorbent towel on the surface is all that is needed to clean up easily.

Diaper-free play often becomes a very enjoyable and vocal part of Baby's day. After diaper changes and after baths are good times to try it. The benefits of some diaper-free time are significant. It provides Baby the chance to feel and move her hip joints without impediment. Moving these joints helps activate the reflexes that support Baby's hips in getting strong for movement. Certain developmental stages, particularly belly-crawling, can be easier for Baby to master without a lump between her legs.

Without her diaper, it is easier for Baby to bring her knees together, and to touch and hold her feet for play, comfort, and learning, which are important early supports for Baby's Natural Movement Development.

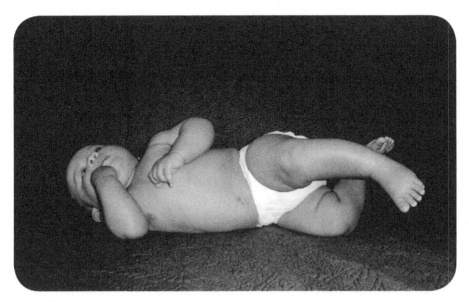

This boy has been rolling for a few weeks. Now when he lies on his side he can feel that he can choose to roll to his back or his tummy.

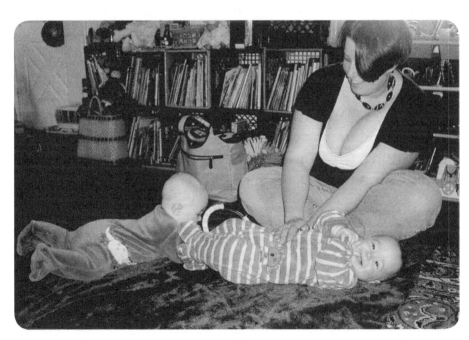

These twins are playing around with rolling.

Rolling from Belly to Back and Back to Belly

When Baby is allowed to play freely on her back, she gets stronger and will start to roll to her side. Sometimes, she twists her head, and her body follows. Sometimes, she turns her pelvis and her head follows. Either way, she will balance on her side or fall forward to her tummy.

After many short tummy sessions, Baby will learn to twist her neck or her pelvis to roll. But before she does this on purpose, she does it a few times accidentally early on. Parents are sometimes baffled that they have seen Baby roll, but then they have not seen her do it again for a while.

Your baby will learn to roll first from her belly to her back or from her back to her belly. Either way, this is an exciting step in her early life.

The In Utero *Position*
Remains the Familiar Side

Whichever side to which Baby's head and spine were curved
in utero will be her more curved side after she is born. She will
look more easily in the direction away from the curve, which is
the way her head has been tucked for some weeks.
Her eye will likely be more open on the side that was less
tucked and one ankle will rest inside the other. I call this the
connective tissue impression.*

This early impression impacts her movement choices. While
it is natural to be more curved to one direction, some babies
resolve this curve more easily than others.

It is possible to soften the intensity of Baby's original curve.
We approach gently and playfully to aid Baby to use her less
familiar side, especially if it helps her fulfill her movement
intention. The goal is not to use each side half the time; rather,
it is to make the less familiar side an accessible movement
choice as she moves toward and away from things.

The connective tissue impression pulls Baby's body in when
she is tired, ill, or during growth spurts. Baby's tendency to
one side is deep and, to some degree, remains throughout life.

Ankles in particular hold the connective tissue impression and
take a long time to mature. The specific way Baby's feet were
tucked *in utero* makes a lasting impression. For everyone, one
ankle is more turned than the other. This is natural sidedness.

(P)ractice

Noticing the Familiar Side

- Baby turns her head to one side more than the other, on back and on belly.

- Baby rolls from back to belly more easily to one side than the other.

- Baby thrusts one leg more than the other.

- Baby mouths one hand more than the other.

- Baby keeps one ankle tucked inside the other at rest.

> I had noticed that my Baby was usually looking to the right, but I had not realized that it was not just her head turned to the right; she also chewed her hand on that side, bent her knee more easily on that side, and rolled to that side when she started to move. It was overwhelming, but exciting, to realize that I could help her use her other side as well!
>
> *A Father*

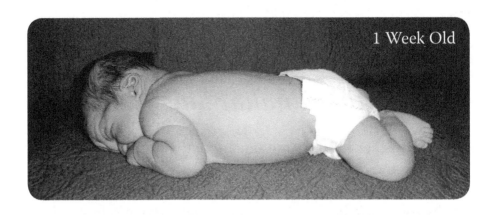

1 Week Old

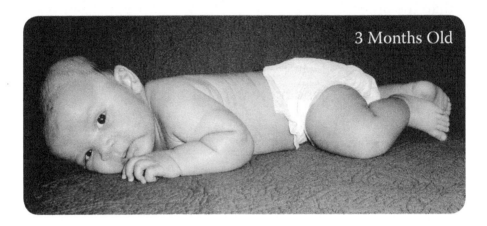

3 Months Old

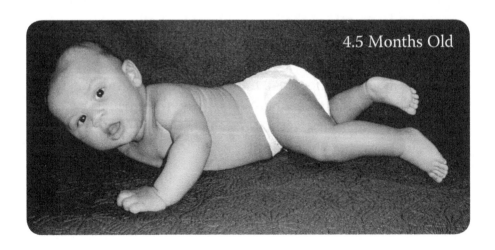

4.5 Months Old

What Having a Familiar
Side Looks Like On the Way

If Baby turns her head more easily to the right while
on her back, she will roll more easily to her right from her
back to her belly. If she lies on her tummy with her head more
often to her left, she will roll more easily to her left from her
tummy to her back.

In belly-crawling, she will be more able to bend her knee
and push with her foot on the side she turns her head to more
easily. When she changes levels from belly-crawling to hands-
and-knees, she will initiate with her right hand to move and sit
back over the left side of her pelvis to sit in play.

If Baby isn't able to belly-crawl or hands-and-knees crawl,
and she does achieve sitting, she may learn to move
forward while sitting by pulling herself along with one leg.

In spinning games, and often in hearing and seeing, she will
feel stronger turning to the right.

It's natural and advantageous for Baby when we create engagement and play on both sides as early as is possible. It starts
with helping Baby learn to look and lie on her left and right
sides with comfort. She will still have a more familiar side, yet
it won't be as dominant (except while learning something new
and challenging) and she'll have easy access to her other side in
movement.

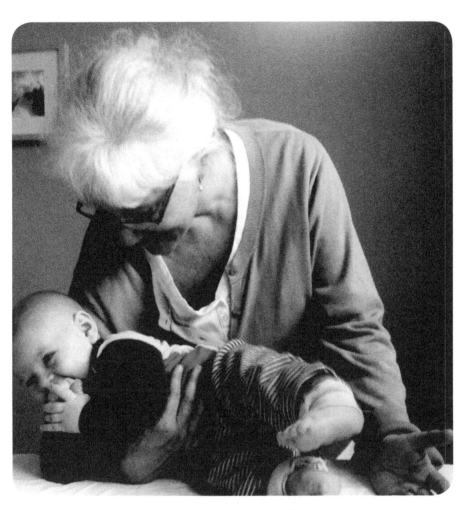

Having fun while building strength on the less familiar side.

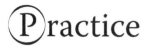ractice

Helping Baby Use Her Less Familiar Side

Start with Baby in her early weeks if possible. If not, start whenever you can.

1. When she is on her tummy, lie down on her left side and her right side and gently call her or hum softly. Give her a chance to turn her head toward what she hears if she is in the mood. Do the same thing sometimes when she is lying on her back.Turning to see what she hears is part of how she learns to roll in both directions. Doing this practice without the diaper gives Baby the full range of sensory opportunities on both sides of her body.

2. Roll Baby onto her tummy or lean her gently onto her more familiar side. Next, roll her toward her less familiar side from back to belly. Then, try rolling her playfully from her belly to her back again on her less familiar side. Once Baby moves in her less familiar direction, let her rest.

3. Let Baby lean out of your lap toward friends and toys. Help her on the familiar side first, then move so that she can lean toward her interest on her less familiar side.

4. Place Baby down on her less familiar side for side-sitting and belly-crawling. Lean Baby into her less familiar hip as you put her down and bend the knee of her top leg.

5. Lean Baby to her less-used side in your lap.

6. Help Baby plant the less-used foot to push up from kneeling to standing.

7. Help Baby get down from standing by dropping her knee down on the less familiar side.

8. When Baby is side-stepping, place enticement at the Baby's less familiar end of the supporting structure.

The familiar side may be obvious to you, or may require careful observation to identify. No worries if you are not sure which side is more or less familiar. Regardless, it is beneficial for Baby when you play with her to her left and to her right, and hold her on both sides of your body.

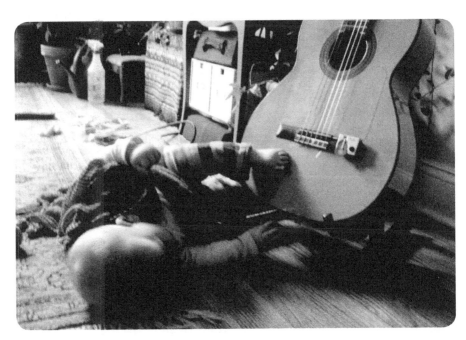

Choose the enticement to Baby's less familiar side carefully!

All Four Sides *Leads to:*

- *optimal, natural reflex opportunities.*
- *a positive foundation for use of all the senses.*
- *a natural relationship to gravity in all positions.*
- *rolling and side-lying.*
- *capacity to play and rest in TummyTime.*

Everything About TummyTime

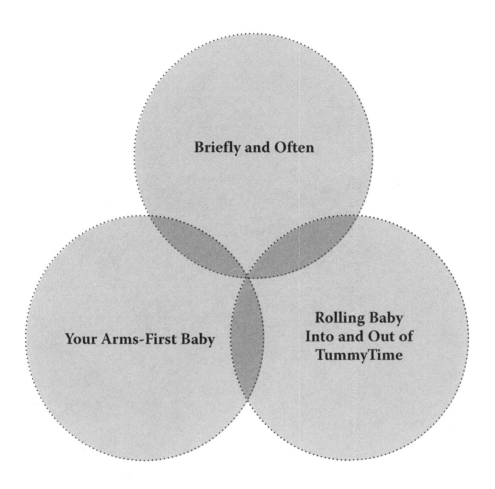

Briefly and Often

Your Arms-First Baby

Rolling Baby
Into and Out of
TummyTime

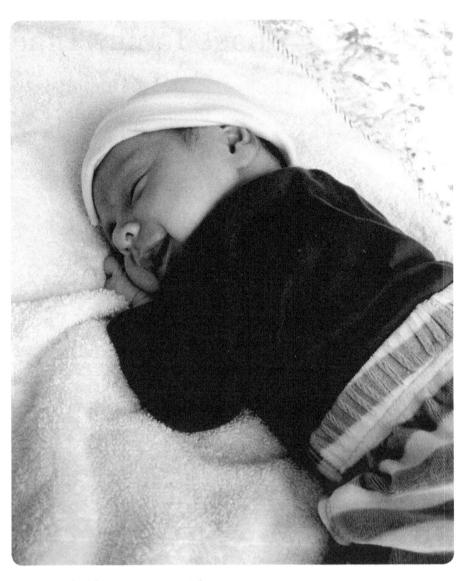

A two-week-old enjoys a private joke.

5. Essentials of TummyTime

Lying on her tummy is an important position for Baby. TummyTime is Baby's foundation for Natural Movement Development. It provides compression to her belly which aids her digestion. It allows her to learn to hold her head up and strengthen her arms. When Baby is on her tummy, she can easily touch or mouth her hands, which soothes her digestion and helps her rest.

TummyTime isn't just good for her; it is the position that provides over fifty percent of the reflex responses that are in her body and brain. These responses provide the skill base for sitting and crawling. Yes, the tummy position naturally engages more than half of Baby's reflex response. These provide a necessary foundation for basic movement and learning skills.

In her earliest weeks, Baby tolerates a few minutes in TummyTime if you are there within sight and reach.

It's ideal to roll Baby off her tummy before she starts to cry, at the first signs of discomfort. This helps her build up strength day by day and week by week, until she can remain comfortably on her tummy for stretches of ten or twenty minutes. Believe it or not, she will eventually roll onto her tummy on purpose when she is finished with breast or bottle-feeding. She wants to play in this position with her toys around her. She has the freedom to move if she chooses.

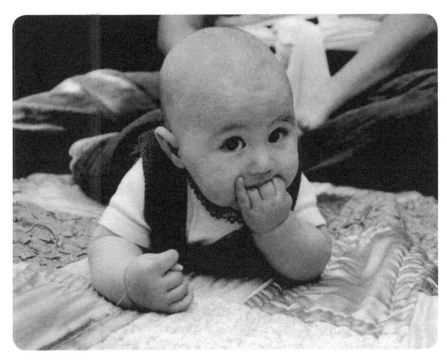

This five-month-old mouths his fingers while observing the camera.

It's Fun Too!

Not only is it good for her brain and body; it's fun.
With each passing week of TummyTime visits, more
and more moments of engaged play occur.

Baby may make more sounds on her tummy, and you may be surprised by her volume. It may seem she's protesting, but usually she's just expressing the new things she's feeling. It's good for her to vocalize, even loudly. Moving more and uttering more go together.

The American Academy of Pediatrics (AAP) recommends: *"Beginning on their first day home from the hospital, or in your family childcare home or center, play and interact with the baby while he is awake and on the tummy two to three periods of time each day for a short period. Place the infant on its belly (3-5 min), increasing the amount of time as the baby shows he enjoys the activity. A great time to do this is following a diaper change or when the baby wakes up from a nap.*

"TummyTime prepares babies for the time when they will be able to slide on their bellies and crawl. As babies grow older and stronger they will need more time on their tummies to build their own strength."

AAP further recommends that you: *"Place yourself or a toy just out of baby's reach so he can reach for you or the toy. Place toys in a circle around the baby so he can develop all his muscles, to roll over, [move]...on his belly, and crawl [on hands-and-knees]."* (Back to Sleep, Tummy to Play, AAP 10/2011).

At first Baby can wobble her head from one side to the other a bit. Often she rests with her head down. Over the weeks in TummyTime, you'll see her learn to hold her head up and look around. She will turn her head to the left and right, holding her head in the middle to look straight ahead with her weight on her forearms. Every time she "stands" on her forearms like this, her neck and arms get stronger, her fists open more, and the range and capacity of her senses expands.

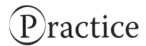ractice

Today Is the Day for TummyTime

If you haven't had a chance to try TummyTime with your Baby yet, don't worry. If Baby has spent some weeks or months lying only on her back, it's okay to try it today.

Remember to keep TummyTime brief. Proceed gently and know that Baby needs repetition over time to get comfortable on her tummy. Stay close to her, preferably on your own tummy or side, and have some fun. Perhaps make faces, goofy noises, or sing. Include a simple, familiar toy if you like.

You may find it remarkable to see Baby peacefully on her belly after her effort to get settled.

TummyTime can become part of ordinary playing no matter when you start. If there are reasons Baby can't practice in her earliest weeks or months, it is truly never too late to introduce TummyTime. Be sure to roll her from lying or tip her slowly from sitting rather than lifting her up and placing her on her tummy. Don't talk about it, just be playful and be sure the visits are brief so Baby does not feel trapped there.

While at first TummyTime might be something you do with a lot of awareness, it becomes an easy part of your everyday life for a long time. Sometimes, even when your baby can move independently, she will choose to rest on her tummy briefly, either on the floor or on you if you are available.

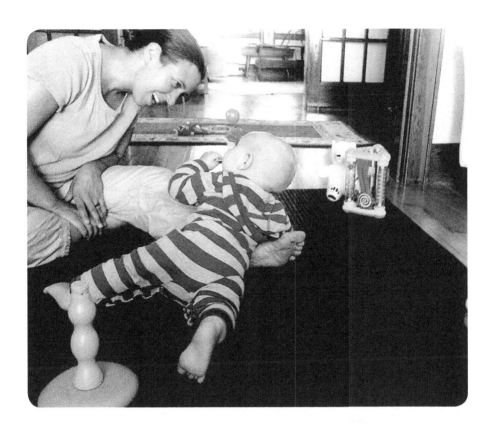

Tried and Cried

Maybe you are reading this and you have already tried TummyTime with Baby, and found that she cried. This can be so discouraging. There are so many good reasons why she might have cried, and why you might have stopped trying. You didn't do anything wrong and neither did she. Use the support of Natural Movement Development to try a fresh start with TummyTime today.

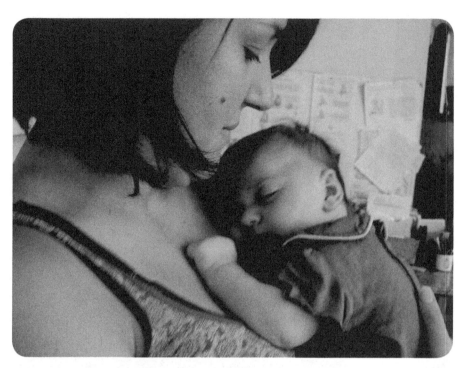

A one-month-old rests on Mom's chest with her forearms by her head.

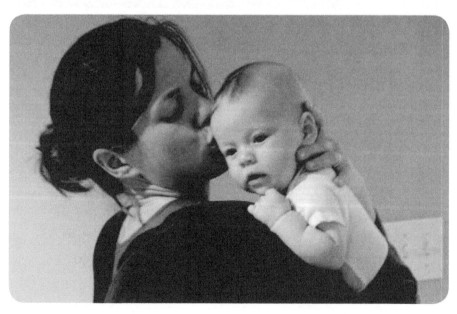

A three-month-old supports herself with her forearms on Mom's shoulder.

ⓅPractice

TummyTime On Your Shoulder

When Baby is held at your shoulder, she's in a similar position to TummyTime on the floor. The difference is that, on the floor, Baby manages her whole body weight, and here you support her weight with your hand under her bottom while she relaxes her upper body into you.

When you hold Baby on your shoulder, check to see if her hands are resting on you near her mouth. If one or both of her arms are hanging down by her sides, help her develop the habit of resting both her forearms on you.

To do so, gently place her forearm against you. Do this a few times a day, until she does it herself. This helps her lift her head to look around when she wants to.

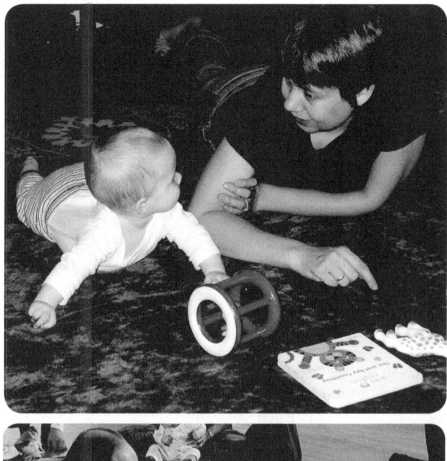

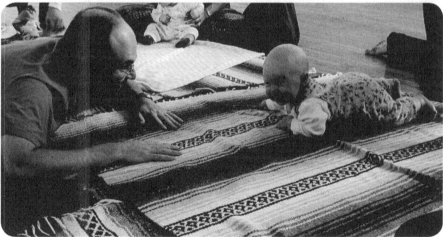

To enjoy TummyTime comfortably together use a firm pad or mat,
covered with a washable blanket. Come ready to play!

(P)ractice

Make a Place for TummyTime

People tell you that your life is going to change when you have a baby, but they don't usually mention your home. Life with Baby means rearranging furniture for years to come.

To nurture healthy development make a special place in your home for it. This is a place for the family to be comfortable on the floor.

TummyTime, and floor time in general, is not just an exercise; it will be a large part of Baby's life and yours: enough to dedicate a space, ideally one where most of your time is spent.

Your coffee table or extra chair might even go to the attic or garage for a year. Start by just pushing it to the side of the room and voila, new side table.

TummyTime goes best for Baby and you when there is an established place in your home for it. A second area, perhaps in the bedroom, is useful too.

Your TummyTime pads can be homemade or store-bought. Refer to the resources section for some of our recommended TummyTime products.

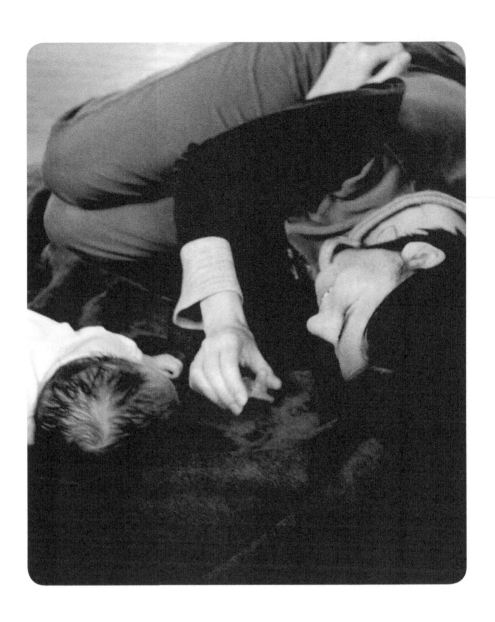

Start with a rug or thick blanket big enough to comfortably accommodate all of you. A pad beneath the rug or blanket is best. Next, throw a washable blanket over the rug. Keep a stack of easy wash-and-dry blankets or towels in a basket nearby.

Or, purchase one of the beautiful washable mats made specifically for TummyTime that are widely available. I also recommend mats made of interlocking foam tiles; these typically remain useful long after TummyTime.

Keep a box of simple and safe toys that Baby can grasp easily. Babies typically put whatever they can hold into their mouths as soon as they are able. This is a part of natural development.

If your dog is the reason you shy away from TummyTime for Baby, consider a playpen. More on playpens in Appendix 3.

Use ordinary activities to provide brief visits to TummyTime, such as after a diaper change.

When you need to put Baby down for a moment, practice making her tummy a go-to choice just as her back is.

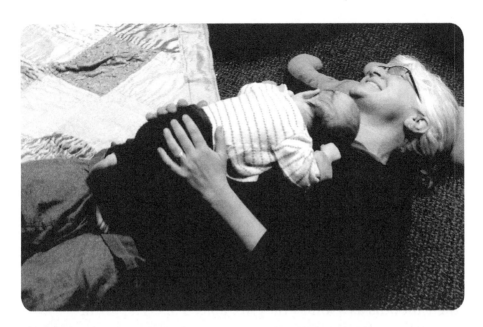

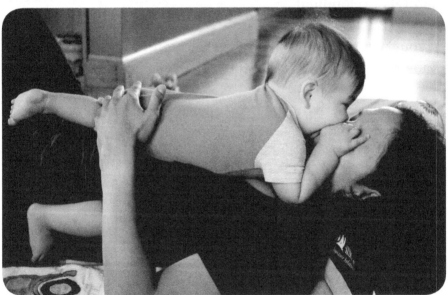

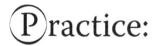ractice:

Tummy to Tummy on You

A wonderful way to help Baby learn to tolerate and then enjoy TummyTime is by laying her on your body. To do so, lie on your back with a pillow under your head. Bring Baby to your chest. Check that her head has clearance under your chin. Once Baby is on you, gently move her arms so that both of her elbows are bent, with her fists by her head. As you can see in the photos, this practice is relevant for a long time; enjoy it with newborns, busy babies, and snuggling toddlers.

Tummy to Tummy supports the bond between Baby and you. You can hear and feel each other's heartbeat. You can feel and hear each other's breath. You can smell each other.

Tummy to Tummy often helps Baby's digestion because it gives gentle, mobile pressure to her abdomen. Tummy to Tummy can be restful—and fun—for both of you.

What's happening here?

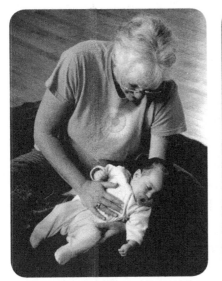
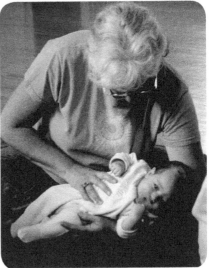

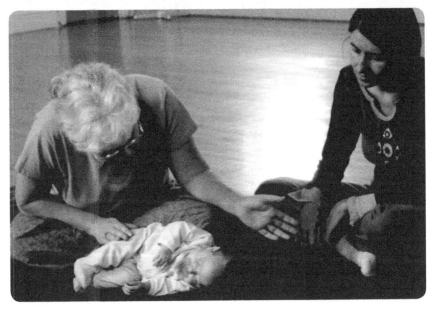

Lenore slides this baby girl from leaning to lying on her side.

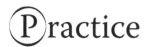ractice

Sliding Baby to the Floor

TummyTime requires repetitive practice in order to become a seamless part of Baby's life. It will be easiest for you both if you can learn to place Baby on her tummy in a way that does not routinely trigger her startle reflex. Frequent startling takes energy, and can be stressful for her. If startling is inadvertently part of your routine it can contribute to Baby's back being stronger than her front. We are trying to help Baby be strong on all her sides, for balance and choice in body and mind.

A practice that may startle Baby when trying to move her to TummyTime is lifting her under her armpits and lowering her, over the tops of her feet, directly onto her tummy. Occasional startling is to be expected—it's part of life. But it is important to know you may be routinely startling Baby as you put her down, so you can find other ways to move her that are less stressful for her.

To do this maintain support behind Baby's head and thighs as you lower her. In her earliest months, lower her toward her side slowly to place her on her hip and shoulder. Let her rest for a moment on her side. Next, gently roll her toward her tummy by tipping her pelvis, not by pulling her arm. This gives Baby time to manage her upper body herself. Each time you do this, look and feel how much more Baby participates and does the movement. It will be one of the many times on the way to walking that Baby works hard to master a movement, and then goes on to do it all the time with ease.

Do As Little As Possible

When you're helping Baby with Natural Movement Development, do as little as possible within each practice. Try to notice which parts of the movement she can do herself, and those she needs you to help with. This keeps changing as you continue to assist Baby to build the skills that help her to regulate and to grow her next independent movement.

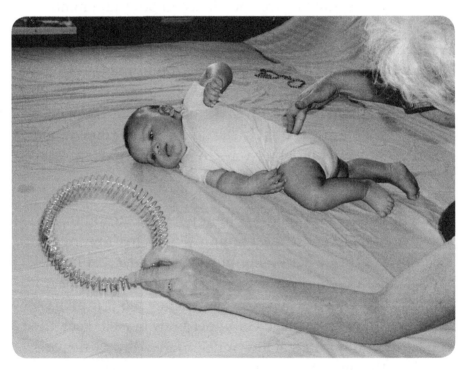

Lenore uses the "one-finger-method" to help this boy fulfill his intention to reach for the toy and roll towards it.

From Back to TummyTime

How Baby gets in to and out of TummyTime affects how well she can settle once she gets there. That is why I teach every parent how to roll Baby from her back to her belly.

Baby will always get plenty of time on her back because that is where she get's her diaper changes, her sleep, and much of her personal interaction.

As Baby has growth spurts, her body sometimes becomes tighter. It is as if the bones have grown and now the soft tissue has to stretch and catch up. For this reason, no matter how well your baby is able to roll from back to belly, she may sometimes grow a bit and seem stuck on her back again. If you observe this, try offering something enticing to her top hand with one of your hands while you gently tip her pelvis towards her interest with your other hand.

Baby's arm is stretched back while she is trying to roll and reach over. This stretch might be a little uncomfortable, but is part of what engages the reflex response which helps her move her arm over. Sometimes, Baby needs a light touch on her hip, briefly, or a tap on her hand. After doing this a few days, she will likely move her top arm freely to roll over in either direction.

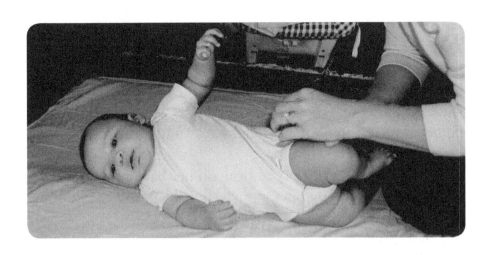

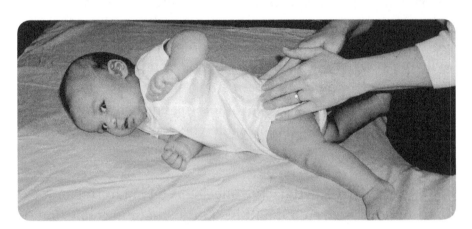

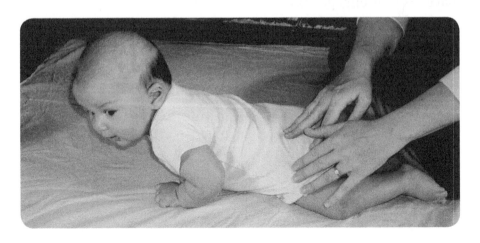

(P)ractice:

Tipping Baby by Her Pelvis from Her Side to Her Tummy

When Baby is lying on her back and becomes interested in something to her side, notice how she tries to roll toward it. Sometimes she can not bring her arm across her body.

Let Baby feel the stretch and then help before she is strained by it. If she is hanging out and not stressed, wait and see if she shows she wants to continue to roll over. Help her by following her interest, tipping her pelvis toward her attention. This is a tiny tip, only enough for her to fulfill her intention of moving to the toy without being stuck by her own arm. Go slowly, remove your hand as soon as Baby takes over the movement toward to the floor.

Whether Baby is plump or tiny, perhaps due to early or stressful birth, in both cases Baby needs this practice. This is because babies are mostly stronger on the back of their bodies than on the front. In other words, Baby's extensor muscles are stronger than her flexor muscles, and so are the reflexes that respond with those muscles. This is a natural part of how we develop. When we help Baby roll easily in both directions—preventing inadvertent falling backward—we help her build essential, natural flexor strength, part of her whole-body skills.

Rolling easily to the left or right on purpose, from back to belly and from belly to back (see pg. 129), builds healthy pathways in Baby's brain and body, positive natural foundations for all her movement skills to come.

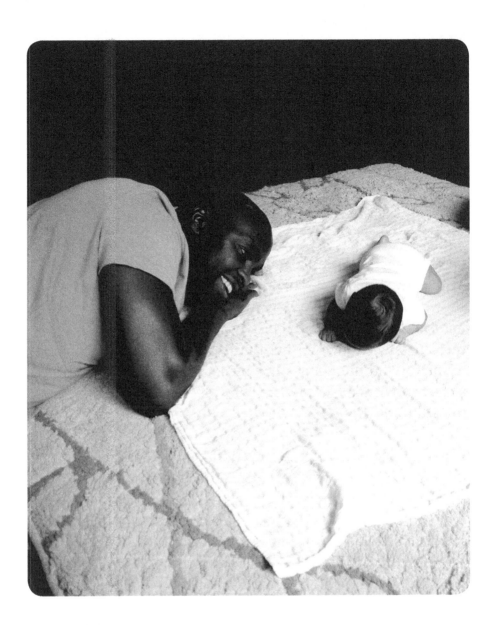

On the Way to Walking

Try It Yourself

TummyTime Together

Make sure there is enough room for both of you to lie comfortably. Lower yourself slowly and be conscious of your back as you lift your head. Only lift your head as far as you are comfortable, without stressing your low back. Feel the skin of your forearms on the floor. Push them into the floor as you lift your head and lengthen your spine and neck. You may tolerate this position for only a few seconds, but that is great! Lower your head to one side or the other to prevent straining your low back.

Baby will lower her head when she is tired. Follow her good example by trying to move as she moves and rest as she rests.

Finish with your practice before Baby becomes tired. Move off your belly by tucking one elbow and rolling over to your side, then to your back. Next, roll again to your side and use your bottom arm to push yourself up to sitting. Let your legs bend to one side as you move up to side-sitting. Next bring your bottom over your heels to kneel. Rest here. Next, place one foot on the floor and push up to stand. Congratulations! you have just moved through the developmental progression. You are awesome! Please pick Baby up and enjoy her in a ball. Rest together.

Ⓟractice

Tucking Baby's Elbow To Roll Out of TummyTime

You will likely see Baby become more comfortable in TummyTime with each passing week. A key to this comfort is your picking her up as soon as she shows signs of tiredness. Try not to pick her up out of habit. Let her stay there as long as she is happily busy or comfortably resting.

When Baby does show signs of tiredness, get ready to roll her off her belly by tucking her elbow. Start by noticing which arm she is facing. Place your hand on the other arm. If Baby's arm is bent, tuck her forearm under her body.

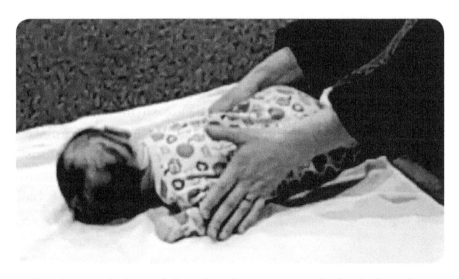

This three-week-old gets help tucking her bent arm under her body so she can roll from her belly to her side.

By four to six months, Baby's arm may be straight by her head when she's on her tummy, not as bent as earlier. If so, tuck her arm under the side of her head. Keep tucking her arm as she rolls from her belly to her side or all the way to her back. These are the movements she uses later to roll independently.

Baby will roll more easily to one side than the other. Note which direction she most often turns her head when lying on her tummy.

Once you and Baby are tucking the arm on the easier side, you are ready to try tucking and rolling Baby to her less familiar side. This practice requires careful thinking at first, and then you both get used to it. Eventually, Baby does it on her own.

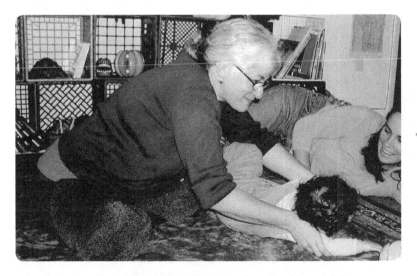

This four-month-old gets help rolling over her shoulder with her arm long to move from her belly to her side.

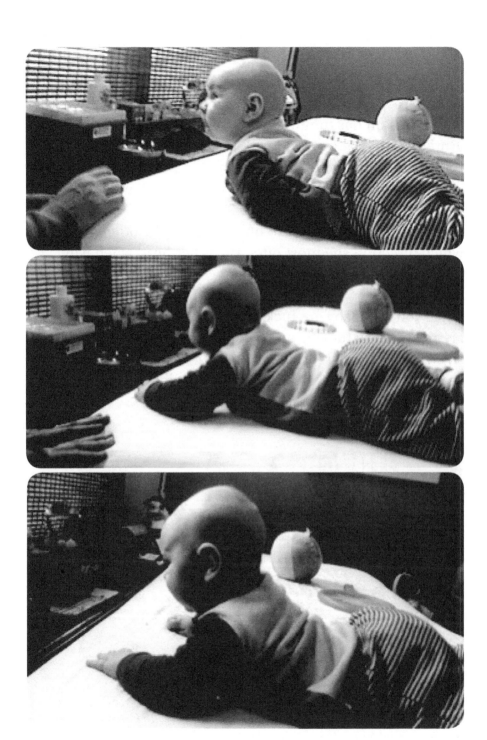

Waiting and watching while Baby frees his arm himself.

(P)ractice

Freeing Baby's Stuck Arm

It is natural for Baby's arm to get caught under her body when she is first learning to roll from her back to her belly. This is not painful for her, although she likely will want to get her arm out. Wait and watch to see what she does.

Of course you will want to help her get the arm unstuck! This practice asks you to briefly hold that urge to free Baby's arm for her. If she is not crying, don't do anything. You are giving her a chance to move her body to build the strength to get her arm free.

If she becomes frustrated:

1. Lift her pelvis on that side just a little bit. Wait and watch.
2. If that doesn't cause her to free the arm, lift the shoulder a tiny bit on that side. Wait and watch.
3. If the above still doesn't help her free her arm, then lift her pelvis on that side a little, use your other hand to move her hand out from under her body and leave her arm there lying by her side. Once again, wait and watch.
4. If she still doesn't bring her hand up by her head, try lifting her pelvis on that side again.
5. If she still does not lift and place her arm, then gently and slowly do it for her. Slowly brush her hand along the blanket an inch or two so that she feels her arm moving and her position change. Repeat with pauses, leaving time for her to move, until her hand rests by her face.

Watch and Wait

When Baby is fresh, let her free her arm herself. If she is tired or has already done a lot today, then free the arm for her. There is no urgency for you or her to get anything right. It is your call, as a parent, as to what is going to be most comfortable for both of you. While it can be challenging to refrain from pulling Baby's arm out for her, the efforts she makes to release it herself are all reflex-driven, from rocking her pelvis off her hand to pulling her arm out and placing it by her head. The more you let her do this on her own at first, the less either one of you will have to think about it later because she will be an expert. She will do it easily with the support of her reflexes. On the other hand, if you help baby without giving her a chance to free her arm herself, you deprive her of the reflex stimulation she needs to become strong and comfortable on her tummy. This is where every baby's foundation of strength lies.

> 〝〝 It would seem so simplistic—too simplistic--to say the best single habit I formed for my younger two kids was to put them on their tummies, but in fact, this is the truth (and they are in second and seventh grades). Tummies gave them time to explore their first year(s) on their own terms and me time to watch them do it—they got more comfortable with exploration and I got more comfortable with both their timetables and their emerging daringness. I didn't feel afraid, because I'd spent enough time with them learning to move to trust them. I think this trust has lasted (so far) their entire lives to date: both ski, one skateboards, and one is on the gymnastics team--and I'm happily awed. 〞〞

Mother of two boys

Football Hold is Not TummyTime

Sometimes Baby is comforted when you hold her under her belly with your forearm, which is called a football hold. You can move her around and she has a good view. The pressure of your arm into her belly can sooth her digestion, so it's one position to try when Baby is gassy. Note, however, that the football hold is not TummyTime. Baby still needs play positions that allow her to bear weight in her forearms.

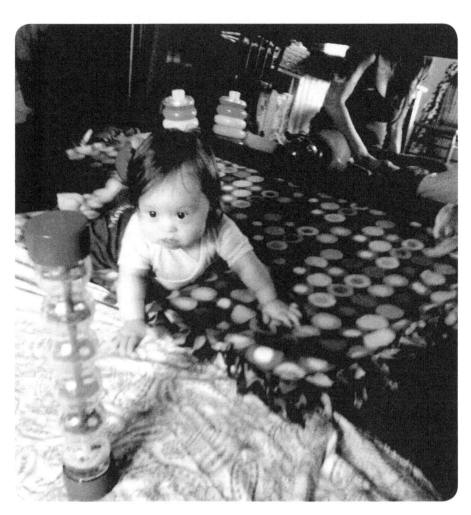

Fascination helps the arms grow stronger.

A Review of TummyTime Essentials

- Make a place for TummyTime.

- Take Baby's socks off before you start.

- Lower Baby to TummyTime arms-first to the floor

- Stay connected: keep physical or eye contact.

- Keep it brief and pick her up before she gets tired.

- Practice tummy-to-tummy with Baby on your body.

- Roll Baby into TummyTime from her back by her pelvis;
  roll her from her tummy to her side or back by
  tucking her elbow.

- Help Baby learn to free her arm herself.

- Keep Baby's neck slightly bent when moving her to avoid
  startling her if possible.

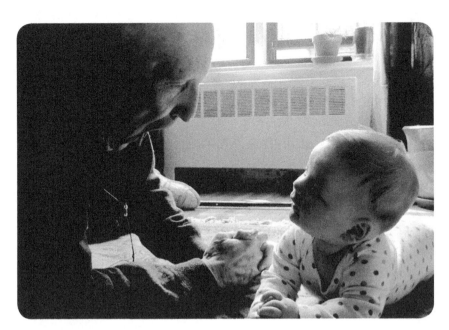

"You're funny!"

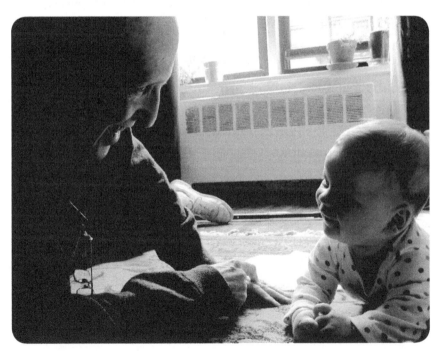

"You're funny too!"

TummyTime *Leads to:*

- *the TummyTime lifestyle and everything in the coming chapters!*

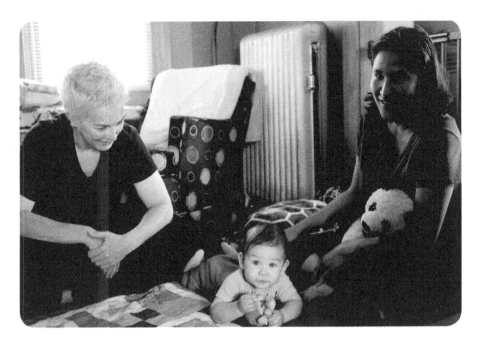

A seven-month-old presides over TummyTime.

6. The TummyTime Lifestyle

Welcome to the TummyTime lifestyle. It is an essential part of Natural Movement Development.

The TummyTime lifestyle starts with brief visits as part of your regular activities. Have one or more TummyTime places set up so that it is easy for you and Baby to catch a moment or two to visit there.

Find a time in your routine that works for both of you. Perhaps after nursing and burping, or after bath time. Maybe the morning is nice after nursing, stretching out on your back in the TummyTime space you've made. Start with Baby resting on you, then let him slide, arms first, off you to his tummy. Keep him company. Lie on your side next to him with a pillow under your head.

Let Baby keep his hands in his mouth when he is on his tummy. Be sure to let him take a break and roll to his side or pick him up before he becomes upset.

If Baby can't settle here, take a break. Then try again, staying close and stopping before he is distressed, if possible. Many babies spit up while on their tummy. This is natural and not a sign that the position is harmful to his digestion. As he gets stronger on his tummy, he will spit up less. If he does spit up, move him to a dry spot or put down a new towel.

In the beginning the length of time of the tummy visit is not the essential part. Short, stress-free repetitions will lead him to extended periods of comfortable TummyTime.

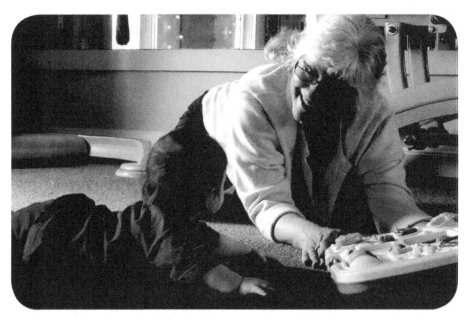

This baby builds strength in TummyTime with interesting company.

❝ The shape of my first son's head was beautiful, he would get compliments on it! I had heard about misshapen heads and wanted to keep that from happening. I wanted to put him in TummyTime because I knew it would help his head stay round, but I found it difficult because he often cried. It wasn't until I became clear that I could pick him up before he cried, that I was able to offer it to him regularly. I needed this reassurance again with my second. It is amazing how much I forgot between the two! The important part was offering TummyTime, not the length of the session. ❞

Mother of two boys

Sock-Free Play

For a baby, socks can be like gloves. It's likely you wouldn't have Baby wear gloves for long stretches of time because he can't feel as much that way. Parents who begin to take Baby's socks off more often report important changes. They mention he moves more when his socks are off and he clearly enjoys his own feet. He plays with them and mouths them when he can, often making sounds. And he gets more traction for the movements he will be learning.

You might be hesitant to take off Baby's socks, concerned that he may get cold. If your feet are not cold in the home, Baby will be warm and safe with his feet exposed for brief play.

It's also ideal for him to be barefoot when feeding sometimes. This gives all his nerve endings the opportunity to develop with natural stimulation: your skin and warmth, the fabric, and the air. Over time he learns to feel all his parts as parts of himself. He will likely learn to play with his feet while lying on his back. (He'll start with one foot being easier to find than the other.)

Bare feet are important for Baby during TummyTime. The sensory input to the skin of his feet increases his possibilities to learn to roll and then to belly-crawl which are the natural movements coming up. A large area of Baby's brain learns from what his feet feel. In adults the ratio of feet-to-brain input becomes smaller than in infancy yet remains important. If you feel comfortable, try it yourself. Take your socks off for a little play-time with Baby.

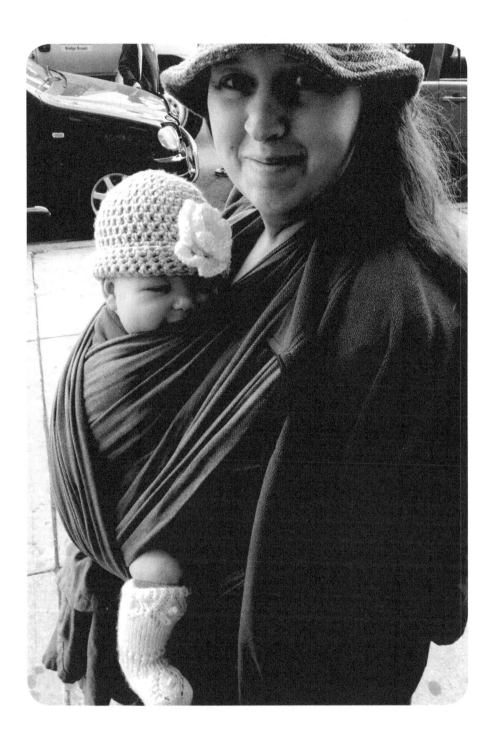

On the Way to Walking

Mouthing is Natural

Baby loves to mouth his hand and, increasingly, he'll put objects in his mouth. This is an important part of how he learns about the physical world. With his mouth and his hands, he explores texture, temperature, shapes, weight, and taste. Putting safe things in his mouth is a healthy response to his environment and a positive developmental activity. Some babies have already been bringing their fists to their mouths *in utero*, others have to learn to connect their hands with their mouths after they are born.

When mouthing, Baby has opportunities to relax, use his hands, and even make sounds in preparation for speech. He may also help himself with teething by putting things in his mouth.

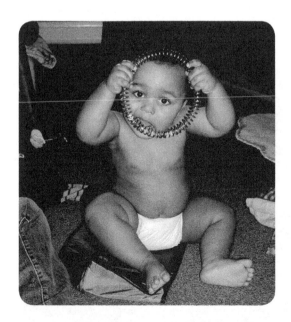

“ I like to have things in my mouth — it helps me calm myself. My mouth and my brain are working together a lot now. I learn how things feel with my mouth. My parents ask me if it tastes good, but really I get more information about texture, temperature, and weight than I do about taste. When I mouth something, I might get all drooly! I don't try to eat the stuff (although it can happen, which is why I'm glad my parents keep small things away from me). Mouthing helps me to manage my stimulating, interesting day. Also, I have a lot of teeth to get through my gums over the coming months, so the more I can mouth things while that happens, the better! ”

Speaking for Baby

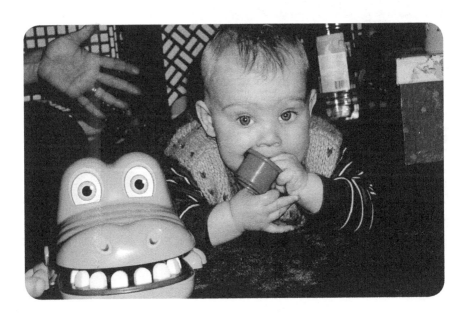

Try It Yourself

Lie Down and Mouth Something

Choose something clean and free of scent to mouth. It can be a book, a bracelet, or a small rattle. Your fist will do as well.

Bring your item with you, lie down somewhere comfortable on your left or right side with a pillow for your head, or on your tummy with your face turned to either side. Bring the object to your mouth with your hand. Hold it in your mouth so that you can breathe comfortably. Explore it with your tongue, teeth, and lips.

Next let the object rest in your mouth while you rest. Let your neck bend just slightly toward your belly. Breathe easily and let your mind quiet for a few minutes.

> " Hey Mama, I made a bitey station for the baby! Will you put Baby down so I can play with him? I found some toys that are good for him to mouth. We can both be on our tummies at the bitey station. If we make a few then I can play with him in every room! "
>
> *Three-year-old boy to his Mom*

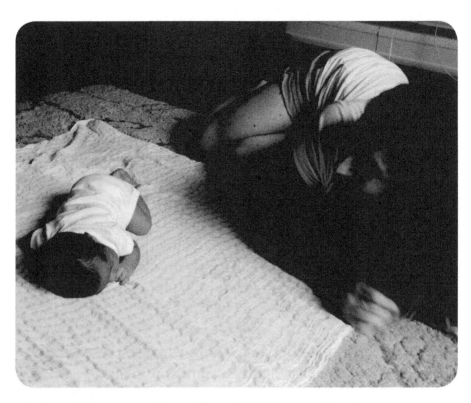

Baby and Mom visit in TummyTime while Baby mouths her fist.

ⓅPractice

Arms Bent for Earliest TummyTime

After Baby rolls into TummyTime and has freed his stuck arm, he might need help to get into his natural movement position. The natural position is with his elbows bent, his hands near his head. Particularly in the first weeks, he may need assistance to activate the response to bring his hand from his side to near his head.

When Baby is new to TummyTime, one of his arms may remain down by his hip after rolling over. Slowly and gently, lift this hip off the floor a little and wait for his brain and body to respond. He'll move his hand up by his head if you give him time. If he doesn't respond when you lift his hip, gently bend his elbow and bring his hand near his mouth.

After a few days or weeks with your help, Baby learns to move his arm himself and will do it independently without need for help. Resting on his tummy, with his arms bent beside his head, allows appropriate development of his *hand-to-mouth reflex**.

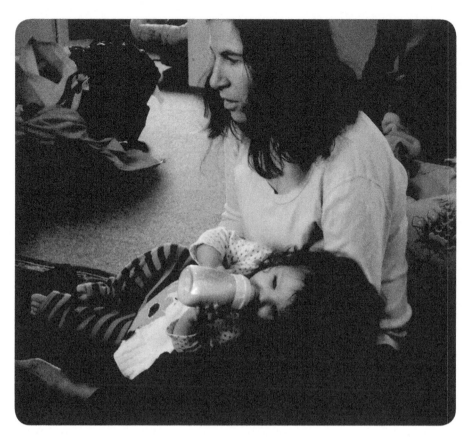

Nursing and bottle-feeding can be restful times in side-lying.

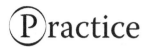

Practice

Letting Baby Rest on His Side on You

This simple practice is a fundamental investment in the natural reflexes for which Baby's brain and body are designed. It can be done when the Baby is swaddled or unswaddled. Ideally, it will be one of the many natural ways you hold Baby through his first year and beyond.

Resting while lying on each side is valuable for Baby. It helps his reflexes to engage naturally and optimally in the coming months.

Try it in the few relaxed moments when you are sitting together. This will be helpful to practice if you have a second Baby and your first is now a busy toddler or young child.

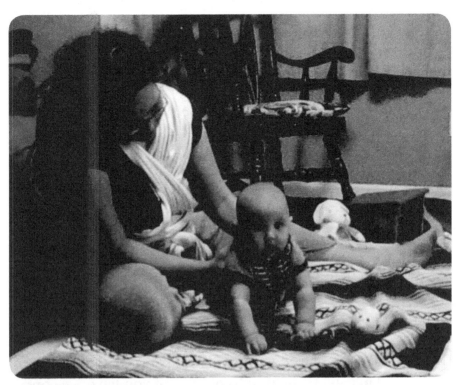

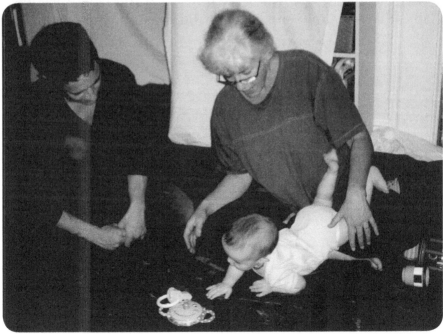

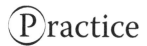ractice

Your Arms-First Baby: Protective Extension

*Protective extension** is an essential reflex for protecting ourselves with our hands and arms when we feel ourselves falling. You've probably done it hundreds of times without thinking. If you start to fall, you thrust your hands out to protect your head.

When moving Baby from one place to another, give him a chance to anticipate the destination with his arms in protective extension. Take care not to cover his arms with your arms when moving him arms first to his tummy.

Protective extension is natural and is something to fertilize through your awareness as you hold and move Baby. The strength of Baby's protective extension is growing through infancy and childhood. Baby builds this strength through rolling, tipping, stumbling, and falling while playing.

At first, with your newborn and very young baby, rolling in to and out of TummyTime comes first. As your baby gets bigger and is aware that he wants to go to his tummy, you can lower him so that his arms are free. Guide his pelvis to the floor as he reaches out to land on his hands or forearms.

It begins with early leaning in your lap. Hold him by his waist and help him tip safely toward the receiving surface, in this case the floor. He doesn't need to get all the way there on the first try. It's helpful for him to tip comfortably, even if he makes only a small motion toward the floor. His brain and body are learning to put his arms out to protect his face.

At first, Baby's response is small. With each passing month, he uses his arms to anticipate the floor to protect his head more and more. This continues as Baby becomes a more wiggly, active person.

When we are at our maximum in learning or working, we will likely be leaning into our most familiar position. Our low brain brings us to our most organized body position to support what we are trying to do and to help keep our energy focused. We go down the most familiar road so that we have more energy to put towards our focus.

It is natural if Baby has asymmetry in his body, and his movement choices; this is just what nature does. We are each asymmetrical, more so in some areas of the body than others. Much of Baby's early body asymmetry becomes less obvious, yet some remains. Most of us feel stronger and more organized on one side of the body than on the other.

If you want to help Baby use his less familiar side, it's essential to understand that he still may not use that side as a first choice. But, he may let you place him there more easily over the days and weeks that you practice, and he may play there briefly before shifting back to his familiar position. This is good for Baby's brain and body and does not mean you are not doing enough. The result of the practices will vary: some babies will be noticeably more bilateral, and others will continue to predominantly use the familiar side although they absorb the practice with increasing ease.

Taking Care Along the Way

When your baby reverts to his more familiar side, that does not mean anything negative about you or Baby. If you have been trying these practices, it doesn't mean they are not working. Some babies (later people like us) have deep familiarity on one side. It is just so good to know that when they are fresh you can play with them on the less familiar side and put them down in the less familiar way and put the toy to the less familiar direction. This can be done once a day—not all the time—so you and Baby can keep practice to the less familiar simple.

Try It Yourself

Lie down comfortably on the floor on your tummy. Notice which side your nose is pointing. Now sit up and notice which arm you used more to push up. Now slowly put your hand on a supporting table or sturdy chair and pull yourself up to standing. Which arm did you put on the table and which foot did you put on the floor to push up? Now observe which side you used in each of the above exercises and whether or not they feel related.

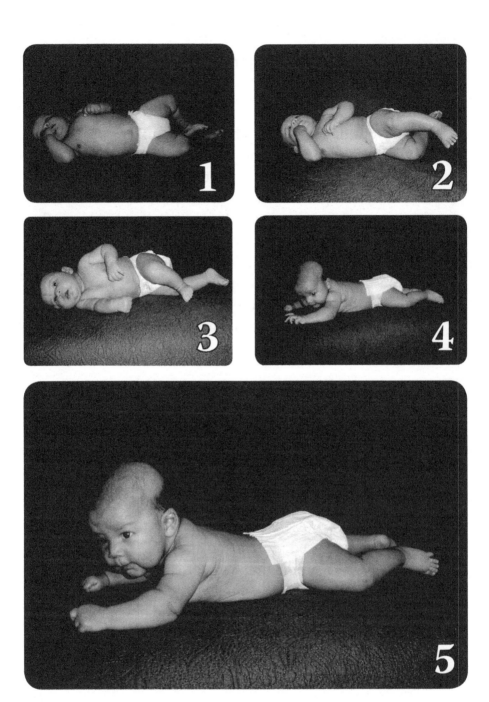

This baby boy rolls over by moving his neck, then his hips, followed by his top leg, and lastly his top arm.

Independent Rolling

Rolling is fun for Baby. And it is natural. It triggers brain development just at the time the brain is ready for it, to feel the pull of gravity in all directions, and to feel himself rolling from one place in space to another.

If Baby spends time on his tummy, he'll turn his head to look around, to follow his interest with his eyes. After he's been on his tummy some weeks, when he follows with his eyes, his head turns too, and this twists his neck a bit. This twist activates reflexes low in his brain that say, "Neck is twisting, follow with body!" And so he does.

In the best case, what I call the *safe small fall** occurs. Baby is not upset, does not even cry, although he falls from his belly to his back. Sometimes parents see this initial rolling only once or a few times and then not again until days or weeks later. Then he starts to roll from belly to back on purpose because his brain and body know how.

After rolling, sometimes Baby has some difficultly managing the weight of his head. Then his reflexes engage to lift his head with support from his forearms.

After several tries, you will see him do it with more ease, rolling off his belly using his muscles so that he does not bump his head. He can choose to remain in side-lying, which he enjoys doing as it affords a 180 degree view.

Some babies roll first from their backs to their bellies. This is fine too! The same kind of reflexes help make it happen. He follows something with his eyes and head, his neck twists, and his brain tells his body to follow his head - and over he goes!

Tucking Baby's elbow when on his tummy, described in the TummyTime chapter on pg. 162, provides the essential stimulation for the reflex response he needs in order to learn to roll independently. Knowing this, you can make it easier for Baby to enjoy TummyTime because he knows with his body experience that he can roll over when he is done.

Rolling increases communication between Baby's brain halves. This is the foundation for belly-crawling, which is harder for Baby to achieve if he does not roll first. However, it is never too late to try rolling play with Baby.

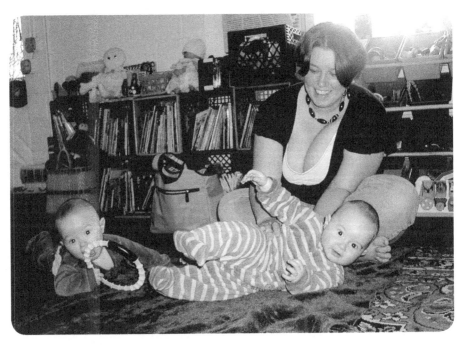

Mom playing with her rolling twins!

Locomotive Rolling

Some babies roll in just one direction. Some roll in both directions, back to belly and belly to back. A few roll more than one time in one direction and end up moving through space on the floor. This is locomotive rolling.

The benefit is the fun and excitement of movement for Baby. The challenge, when the time comes, will be shifting from moving left or right, to finding the push in the arms and legs to go backward or forward. If you notice that Baby is interested in something and rolls away from it, this is an indication to explore the practices in the belly-crawling section.

Rolling is Baby's first independent movement in space. Babies may roll from belly to back first or back to belly. Once Baby starts to roll in one direction, playfully roll him to both directions once or twice a day until he can go both ways independently.

Startle and Recovery On The Way

Startling is information. It tells Baby if he is falling or getting too much sensory information at once. Small startles during movement build muscle tone as Baby works to regain his balance. This is what happens in the pictures below.

Occasional startling helps Baby learn to recover. These are the safe small falls which build physical and psychological confidence and resilience.

The seven-month-old we see below heard me come in and looked up from his play to greet me as I photographed him. He reached towards me with enthusiasm, causing the muscles on the back of his body to engage, making him tip back unintentionally.

When he felt this, his reflexes brought his arm forward again so he could protect himself from rolling all the way back. His weeks of playful rolling practice helped him to flex his limbs forward to recover his comfort on his tummy.

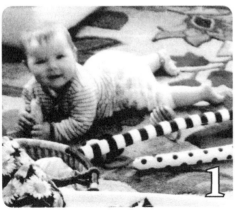 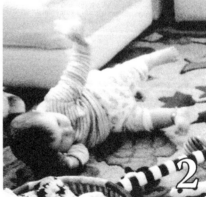

Try It Yourself

Recover from Startle

Startle and recovery is a part of everyday. It starts *in utero* and continues through our lives. Startle happens, and regrouping from startle happens.

Baby has to manage the unexpected and his reaction to it, and so do we. Recovery from startle is personal. Please explore gently.

Think of something that concerns you and allow your back to tighten and your arms to pull back to demonstrate your concern.

Now, gently consider coming into the present and telling yourself that there will be a way to meet this concern. Allow your back to soften and your front to engage. Let your face drop toward your chest until you feel calm.

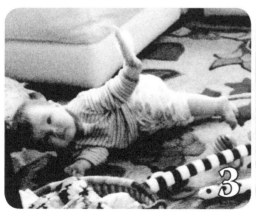
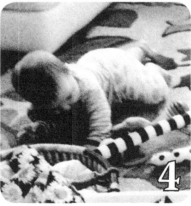

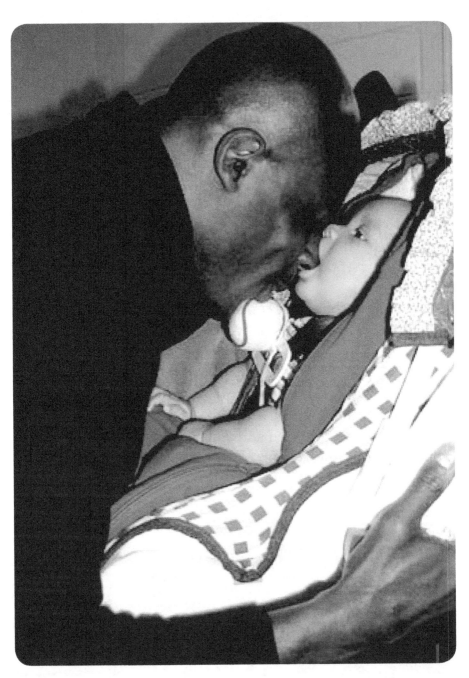

Father and son share good times in the car seat.

Use the Car Seat for the Car

The portable car seat is a recent piece of equipment in the history of babies. The car seat is essential for Baby in the car, and its purpose is to hold Baby securely in place. However, it restricts Baby's movement and visual field, and long hours over the weeks in this seat can make it difficult for him to feel comfortable in natural TummyTime play.

Take some time to associate the car seat with loving play. Keep one or two toys attached. If Baby is asleep in his car seat upon arrival at your destination, you might choose to leave him in the seat until he wakes. You can also try taking him out of his seat without waking him, having safe places ready such as a hammock, bassinet, floor pad, or playpen.

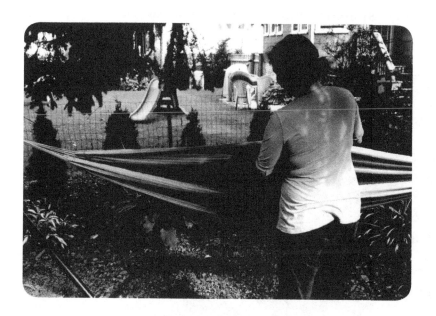

Early Toy Interest

Typically between two and three months of age, Baby will take some interest in basic toys. He'll look at them and make efforts with his arms to grasp them, wanting to touch them and get them in his mouth.

If Baby has digestive discomfort or other stress in his early weeks, his attention may not turn outwardly as much or as soon as if he were more comfortable. Later, in the weeks ahead, his digestion will improve, and his brain and body will grow a little more mature. Then, when he's feeling better, he will focus his attention outwardly more often.

This is a reason why typical developmental time windows for some skills are so broad; motor development slows when Baby's system is addressing other stressors.

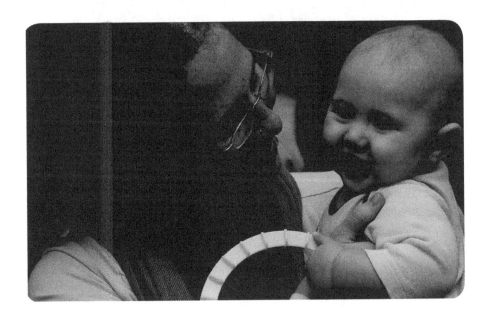

Tips for Back Play

• Hold a toy over Baby's middle and let him practice moving his arms to grab it. You will see him trying long before he can do it accurately.

• Touch each hand with the toy and then bring it back over Baby's middle. Observe him using his arms and hands.

• Avoid using a close-hanging activity center unless you need it for a moment of babysitting safety.

• Hang a mobile or other spinning objects in each area where Baby nurses and plays.

• Gently teach Baby to hold his own bottle over time by bringing one palm and then the other to the bottle and helping him hold it as he eats.

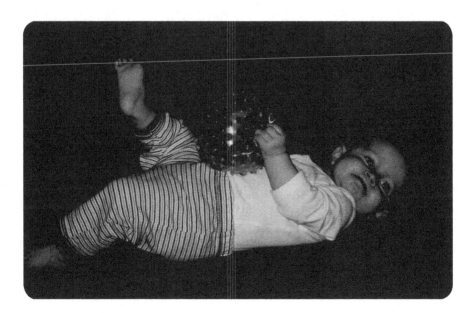

If Baby Does "Sit-Ups" Or Moves Along the Floor on His Back

On his belly, he learns to roll, push back, and crawl forward along the ground in his own unique way. On his back, he learns to look all the way around from one side to the other. Then he learns to hold things in his hands and bring things to his mouth. He often holds his knees, and his feet, which are wonderful built-in playthings for him. When he plays with feet he makes a connection between all his limbs and his mouth. This can provide playful and restful self-regulation. It helps him feel oriented through his whole nervous system. He will learn to roll to one side, and next roll over to his belly.

When Baby plays on his back, he may like to move his legs, bang his heels, or push his feet into the floor, making a bridge of his back.

If he gets in the habit of pushing hard with his legs and feet while on his back, he may start to move along the floor this way, pushing headward with his feet. If you see him moving on his back along the floor this way, it is an indication that he needs help to roll over and find this same pushing action when on his tummy.

It is good that Baby is moving; however moving on his back this way makes it harder for Baby to tolerate being on his Tummy, where he learns to belly-crawl. If you see Baby moving along his back, or lifting his head while he is on his back, looking like he is doing curl-up exercises, it means he is strong enough to learn to move on his belly.

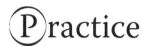ractice

Moving Baby to His Belly

In this practice, you roll Baby from his back to his belly if he's pushing headwards on his back with his legs or doing "sit-ups".

Playfully engage Baby while he is busy on his back. Join him in the excitement of pushing and moving that he is doing. Then place one hand lightly on his far hip and say "I'm going to roll you over". Gently pull his hip, rolling him to his belly as he pushes with his legs, to direct the pushing strength into rolling over instead of into sliding headward along the floor.

Stay with him on his tummy and keep the play going. This allows him to develop most naturally by reaching with his arms and pushing with his legs.

Be sure there are toys within and beyond reach. Follow his interest as you help him to bend one leg or the other, as he tries to move forward. Continue from here with the practices in the belly-crawling section (see pg. 207).

It's not supposed to be perfect. Try it a few times and let Baby roll to his back whenever he wants to.

This practice will need repetition over days. You are helping Baby direct his movement energy where it will feel best to him by rolling him quickly and playfully to his tummy. There is no need to struggle at all. If he doesn't want to stay, let him roll freely to his back. Try again another time.

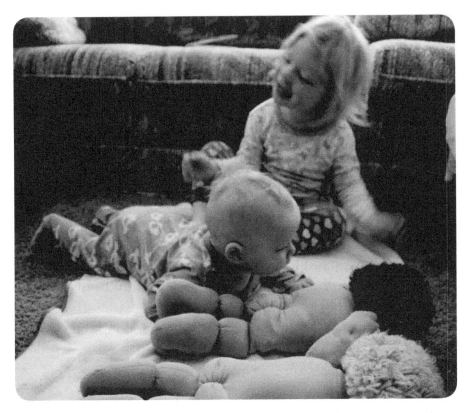

Big sister instructs class for TummyTime participants.

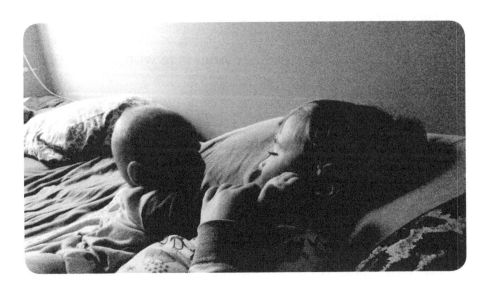

TummyTime with
Your Second Child

It is hard, but it is possible! You can expect that your second child is going to get less TummyTime than your first. No worries! All the benefits he gets from observing his older sibling far outweigh what he misses. Aim for five minutes a day of tummy rest or play for your new one in the first few months and let this time be different.

> " One of my biggest challenges having my second child is how to be sure she has some opportunities for TummyTime each day. My older daughter, two years and two months old, has so much energy and so much affection for her baby sister that this translates into being dangerously rough with her sometimes. Any time I put the baby down, my energy is given to protecting her from her big sister. So I have made the commitment that I will give the baby at least one TummyTime session while my older daughter naps in the afternoon, and another after she goes to bed at night. So at least twice a day the baby will spend some time on her tummy. Lately, as both girls are getting a little older, they've had a few safe sessions of play while the Baby is having TummyTime. "

A mother of two children

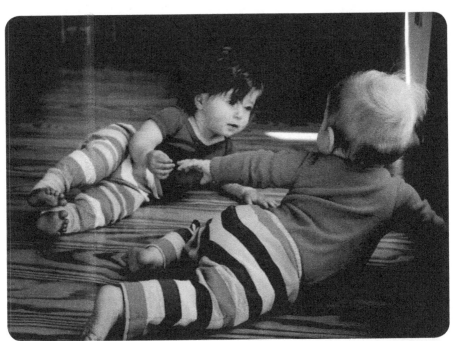

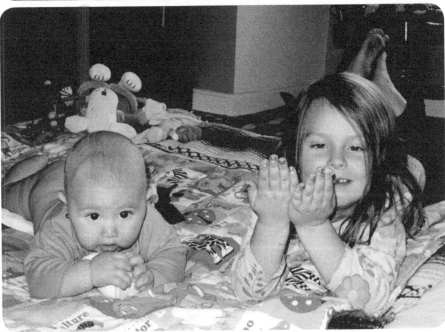

TummyTime with friends.

The Tummy-Time Lifestyle
Leads to:

- *holding his head up while supporting himself on his forearms.*
- *pushing all the way up into long strong arms, then pushing backwards.*
- *making louder sounds.*
- *bringing his hands and objects to his mouth.*
- *pivoting on his belly.*
- *pushing up to sitting.*
- *belly-crawling forward.*
- *Baby moving independently, safely on the floor.*

Starting to Get Around

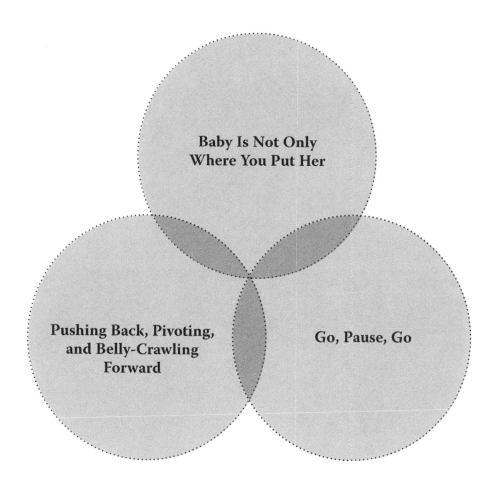

Baby Is Not Only
Where You Put Her

Pushing Back, Pivoting,
and Belly-Crawling
Forward

Go, Pause, Go

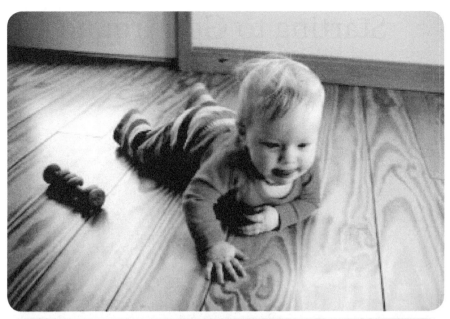

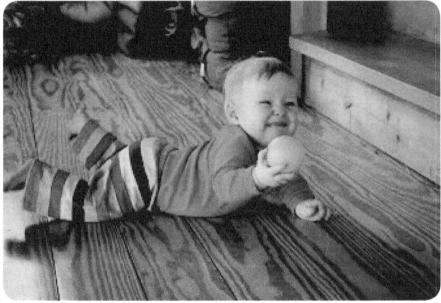

7. Belly-Crawling

Baby begins to move around more, as her desire to explore expands. This can be a bittersweet moment. We wouldn't wish for our children not to belly-crawl, yet it is the end of the most innocent part of infancy. In this new phase you can no longer be sure that you will find Baby where you left her.

Until now, all of Baby's movements, other than rolling, have been interdependent with you.

This notable change for you and Baby is a new chapter in your precious journey together. It feels different to both of you when Baby can move about on her own. She still wants to be held closely in your arms. She's also ready to explore her environment and will spend less time on your body. Baby experiences an expanded understanding of who and where she is as she moves in the world around her.

Ironically, she builds up to moving forward by moving everywhere but forward. She pushes up on her arms, she pushes herself backward on the floor. She may pivot around her belly button to one direction or both. She may even push back so much in her effort to go forward that she pops up onto her hands-and-knees. All these movements are good. They are parts of the whole, which is belly-crawling forward.

Baby has long periods of time playing contentedly on her tummy, during which she learns to bend one knee or the other on the floor. This contented and busy stationary play is a foundation of belly-crawling. Belly-crawling develops as Baby sees and wants things that are out of her reach.

Belly-crawling is advantageous for her brain and body. It is a big step in Baby's development involving new activity across the middle of her brain.

Crawling* is associated with hands-and-knees (confusingly it is called creeping* in academic terminology). But, in fact, when allowed and encouraged, Baby will crawl first on her tummy.

This belly-crawling* is sometimes called commando crawling* or pre-crawling*.

Baby expends a lot of effort learning to belly-crawl. She'll appreciate some help from you, as belly-crawling is complex, and Baby achieves it over time with much practice. Most babies have difficulty when first trying to move forward. They want to move but can't, and they feel frustrated. Ironically, a moment of frustration is often when Baby pushes her foot into the floor and moves herself forward.

To correctly understand how the big toe supports the whole movement, you've got to get down on the floor and try it. But don't think about your toe! Put your attention on something interesting that is out of your reach and move toward it. Your phone perhaps, with an unread text on it?

With repetition Baby will become agile, slithering like a lizard. She'll move readily over your lap, toys, and other obstacles.

Some babies move forward on their bellies by pulling themselves along with their forearms. Other babies move forward by pushing with both feet, like a frog. Both of these look like belly-crawling. It is good for Baby to be moving around. However, if she's doing either of these movements exclusively, and not able to push with one foot and then the other, try to give her a little help. Refer to "Components of Belly-Crawling" on page 209.

Remember, not every baby will be able to do this. Try it, but don't force it. The important thing is for Baby to be moving forward.

Belly-crawling naturally leads to the next, more complex, movement of crawling on hands-and-knees. When allowed to develop naturally and assisted when needed, belly-crawling, as a primary way of getting around, lasts from a few weeks to a few months before Baby progresses to predominantly crawling on hands-and-knees. Parents may hope for hands-and-knees crawling without knowing that belly-crawling exists, let alone that it comes first.

Belly-crawling is demanding for Baby's brain and body. It takes weeks for Baby to figure out. Often there is a stage of pushing backwards. Babies might persist in rolling and need help to push back or reach forward. These movements are easiest for Baby to learn before she moves on her hands-and-knees.

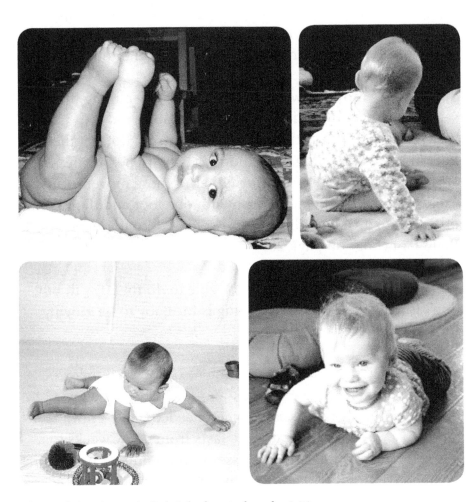

So much is going on in Baby's body, mind, and spirit!

The Parts Work Together
To Make the Whole

Baby is usually working on all these motor skills at the time that belly-crawling is coming together. These skills occur around the same time, and each helps the other, until the pieces become coordinated movement sequences:

• Holding the toes while on her back.
• Supporting herself while side-leaning.
• Moving to sit up from her tummy.
• Moving to the side and then to her tummy from sitting.
• Pushing to slide backwards while in TummyTime.
• Pivoting on her belly button to the left or right while in Tummy-Time.
• Airplane.
• Belly-crawling forward by pushing exclusively with one foot and reaching with the arm on that side.
• Interest in things beyond her reach.
• Wanting to move before she can.

Movement skills in TummyTime build slowly. It can take awhile to get comfortable in TummyTime, and then there an be weeks, even months, of contentment playing here, before Baby's senses, interests and efforts start to perceive and move further into her environment.

Moments of Frustration

As you practice together, Baby becomes comfortable on her tummy. She enjoys it most days and plays there contentedly for a little while, especially if she can see or at least, hear you nearby. As her strength and her distance vision increase, she becomes interested in things beyond the circle of her contentment; then she tries to move toward those things. As Baby grows stronger in TummyTime, she shifts between contentment with what is within reach and her ambition for things beyond reach.

Frustration is part of this moment of development. While learning to belly-crawl, it is actually the experience of frustration that gives Baby the power to push into the new movement. Some babies cry with surprise as this happens, and some do not notice.

A little bit of frustration helps Baby learn to move, while a lot of frustration helps Baby learn to be frustrated. Each parent has to make their own choice here, letting Baby expend her effort sometimes, doing it for her other times, and all the grey area in between.

Teething

Teething is uncomfortable, and it can go on for weeks
or even months. Some days are better than others. Teething
days are teething days. They are days focused on comforting
Baby, rather than all the things you planned, including your
developmental practice. Baby's comfort comes first. Try every
trick in the book to help your baby manage teething.

Keep trying until you find one or more teething objects that
Baby will mouth for relief. It doesn't have to be a teething toy.
For example, Baby might like an ice cube in a washcloth
rubbed on her gums. Ask your friends what worked for their
baby. Cut yourself some slack on Baby's tough teething days.
This is not the best part of being Baby or of parenting.

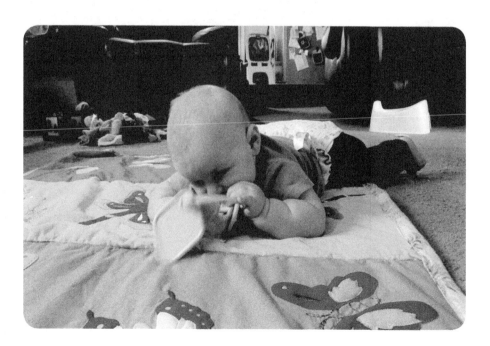

What is happening here?

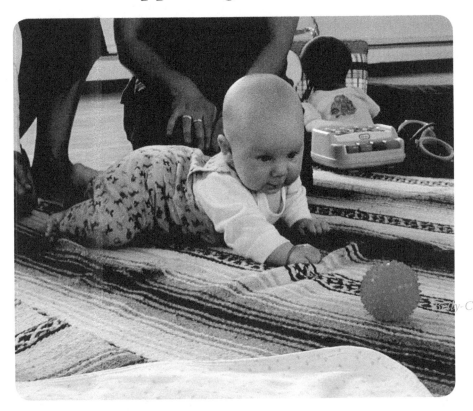

This boy is on the verge of belly-crawling. He doesn't have to do anything. Maybe he is happy looking at the ball and thinking about it. He won't try to move until he is ready. He won't think about moving; he'll just do it when the time and his skills are ripe.

Components of Belly-Crawling

- Begins with Baby reaching with her arm, while in Tummy Time, toward an interest that is out of reach.

- As she reaches, her leg on the reaching side bends at the knee, and her weight rests on the opposite side of her pelvis (weighted side has straight leg).

- The bent leg allows the big toe on that side to make contact with the floor.

- As Baby reaches, she pushes the ball of her big toe against the floor, which slides her whole body forward slightly.

- As she does this, her pelvis tips, causing weight-bearing on the opposite side.

- This weight shift allows her to reach with her other hand. This reaching then bends her knee on that side, which next triggers Baby's reflex to push with the ball of her big toe to move herself forward. Each of these movements is a *belly-crawl step* along the floor.

- Each time she shifts from one side to the other, she becomes more able to use her two sides together, eventually becoming a busy, belly-crawling Baby.

Airplane On The Way
to Belly-Crawling

When Baby gets ready to belly-crawl, a new reflex is engaged. In TummyTime she lifts all her limbs away from the floor with full extension of the back of her body, and then brings her limbs back to the ground. This *Airplane Reflex** (*Landau Reflex**) is similar to the startle reflex, as it also has two phases. It engages a little later in her development, part of nature's plan to help her build strength and momentum to move through space. Similarly to the startle reflex, Baby may do the first phase and be challenged to complete the second phase.

ⓟractice

Releasing Airplane

If the first part of Baby's airplane, the spreading part, is very active, Baby appreciates help a few brief times a day, to playfully complete the second part, returning her limbs to the floor. To help with this, give Baby a hug from behind as you fold her arms and legs down to the floor, then let go. If you've been picking Baby up by her waist, holding her high and pretending she is flying for fun or distraction, try decreasing this practice and see what happens. It is cute and fun, but doing it often at this stage may make Baby's back muscles tight, which makes it harder for her to use her arms and legs to learn to belly-crawl.

$\textcircled{P}$ractice

Sock-Free Especially for Belly-Crawling

It is a big job for Baby to master belly-crawling. She is gaining more movement and emotional skills. Belly-crawling is the first point in motor development in which frustration is a necessary ingredient. Not a lot of frustration, only a moment, usually accompanied by a strong sound or a cry. Bare feet during TummyTime makes all this easier, the skin contact engages Baby's reflex responses and gives her sensory information about her environment. The skin contact with the floor also helps Baby release the spreading part of her airplane response.

Let Baby play with her feet bare on different floor surfaces. You may be surprised how she is more able to belly-crawl on one surface than another.

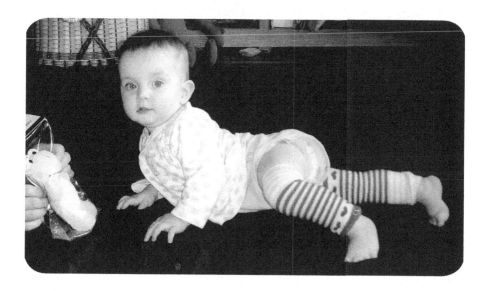

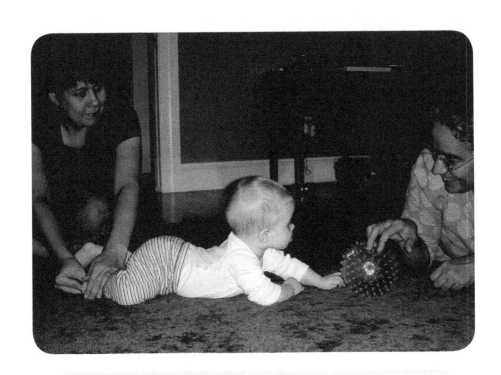

The Essential 45-Degree Angle

Leaning is essential to learning new movements. It can be scary at first—then it's fun! Leaning engages Baby's reflexes for her next stage of movement. Leaning at a 45-degree angle opens new skill sets. When Baby is learning to belly-crawl, place toys at an angle from her line of sight. Learning to tip from side to side is a big step in Baby's maturation. It is necessary in belly-crawling, and makes new connections in her brain and body. She can do more, think and feel more, with increasing complexity.

Ⓟractice

Helping Baby To Belly-Crawl

- Baby's interest comes first. A playful friend with an enticing toy is ideal help for this practice. Baby is not thinking about belly-crawling — she is interested in playing.

- Start by observing which way Baby's head is turned, and whether one leg is more bent than the other.

- Next, place your hand lightly on her shin on the bent leg and rest there. Feel if Baby's leg is resting or active.

- Wait for a moment when you feel her leg muscles soften --this might be brief. That's the moment to bend her knee along the floor, then remove your hand.

- Baby has an easier, more familiar side. It is usually the one she is facing. Bend the knee on the side she is facing.

- Give the ball of Baby's big toe contact with the floor so she can push with her whole leg.

- As soon as you feel her push with her foot, regardless how far she moves, switch to her other leg and bend that knee. If she is content, she will play in place with her leg bent and her arm out. There is no urgency; we help Baby to belly-crawl when we observe that she is trying to move.

- To help Baby bend her more thrusting leg, be ready to move fast. After she bends her familiar knee, immediately bend her other, less familiar leg.

- If you miss your chance, she'll push again with the strong leg. If so, try again in the next cycle to help her bend her tighter leg.

- Be sure to help one leg at a time, not both at once. In other words, help her move like a lizard, not like a frog.

Baby may have difficulty releasing one knee more than the other at first. Over days or weeks, it becomes easier until shifting side to side and bending each knee alternately are a comfortable part of her movement repertoire.

This might feel difficult to do. Just as with TummyTime, don't try too hard or too long, and come back to it again later. If the tight leg does not bend, it does not reflect negatively on you or Baby. Belly-crawling takes practice.

Belly-crawling does not work or look an only one way. Any variation is good. Trying to move around while on her tummy is natural for Baby. It is good for her reflexes, and it helps Baby build more ease of movement. Belly-crawling is typically tough at the start, yet it becomes Baby's way to get around, and builds skills which make later hands-and-knees crawling easier for her. If Baby pops up to hands-and-knees before belly-crawling she will need a longer period of rocking on hands-and-knees, a natural developmental stage, before she can move forward. If she does pop up from her tummy before belly-crawling, please see pg. 216.

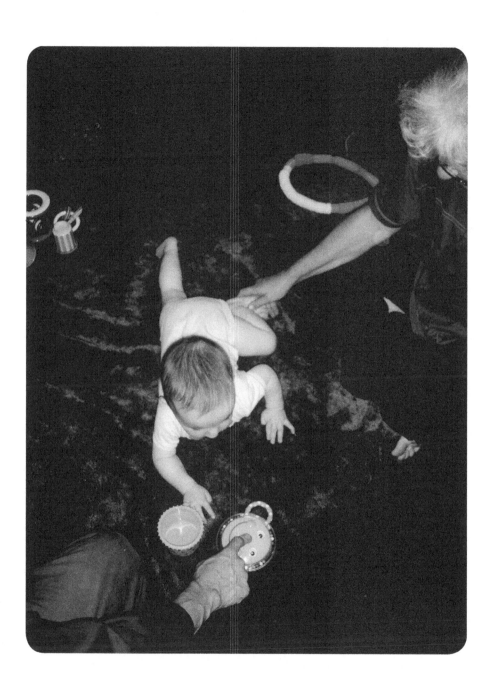

Early Popping Up in Belly-Crawling

If Baby doesn't yet belly-crawl, and she starts to pop up to hands-and-knees during TummyTime, try to bring her body back down occasionally. This may provide chances for belly-crawling pushes before she starts skill-building on hands-and-knees, the next level away from the floor.

Baby might pop up before she can belly-crawl because she has strong thrusting reflexes in her legs. The natural progression of her strength development is for her to support herself on her arms before her legs. This practice helps her build arm strength before she shifts to hands-and-knees.

(P)ractice
Bringing Baby's Pelvis to the Floor

Have a few interesting toys on hand to ensure that Baby has a fun focus while you release her legs down in one of these ways.

1. Place your hand under her belly. Gently pull her knees out to straighten her legs and help the front of her pelvis to rest on the floor.

2. Place your hands under her chest and gently pull her along on the floor until her knees catch and her legs straighten out. Let go as soon as the front of her pelvis touches the floor.

3. If she pops up again, bring her back down again, unless she's tired. Repeat over time, without forcing.

4. Baby may stay down for days, or she may not. You are providing positive opportunities for her brain and body when you bring her down from early hands-and-knees, whether she stays there or not. This is a brief practice: soon Baby will be crawling on hands-and-knees and won't be doing much belly crawling anymore—only in play, when she wants to.

(P)ractice

Letting Baby Rest and Play on Your Lap

When Baby learns to belly-crawl, she'll move away and then crawl back to you during floor-play.

Let her arrive. See if she's visiting or if she needs something before automatically picking her up. This is a new impulse. Until now, your inclination to pick her up is automatic. Now, with increased belly-crawling, she will move away and then back, away and back again. These are exciting explorations for her, and a new dimension of relating with Baby for you.

When you sit on the floor, your body is just the right height for Baby to practice kneeling while she visits you.

This helps her prepare to crawl on hands-and-knees. If you can tolerate it, Baby would like to belly-crawl right over you. Actually, she would like you for her personal jungle-gym along the way.

Belly-Crawling Your Way

Only some babies get all their parts moving evenly and easily for belly-crawling. Every Baby will be a unique lizard!

Belly-crawling has four stages: interest, reach, push, and shift. This is the rhythm of belly-crawling. Try to help Baby find it while also accepting the unique way she does it.

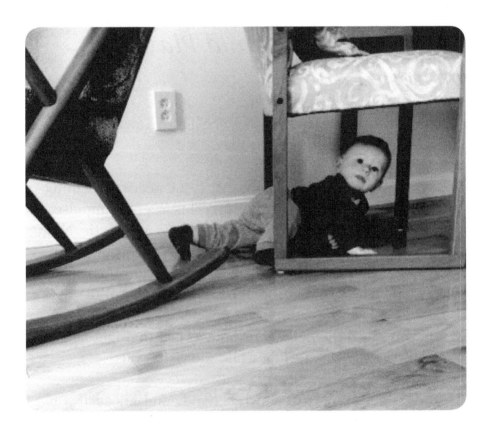

Try It Yourself

Belly-Crawl with Baby

- Get down on the floor and try it yourself.

- Focus on something out of reach.

- Stretch one arm toward it as far as you can go.

- Feel the impulse for your knee to bend.

- Push off with your foot and slide yourself along the floor.

- Feel the natural point at which your other arm wants to reach out and your other foot wants to help by pushing off.

- Try not to think much about what your body is doing. Keep your intent on getting the object of interest that is just out of your reach.

- Let Baby see you practice.

- With attention, you may be surprised at how different your two sides are.

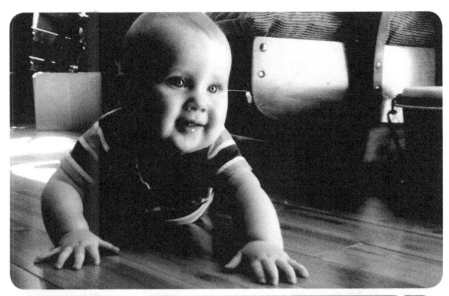

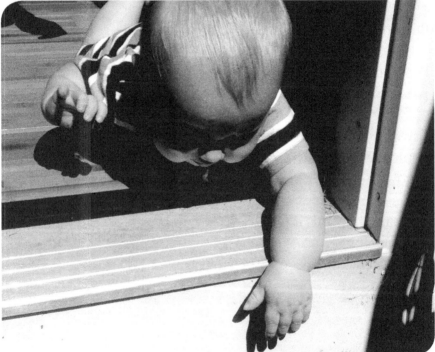

This eight-month-old shows the joy and peril of belly-crawling.

It was wonderful to watch my son learn to belly-crawl! This was a slow process and took place over a 6-week period. Each piece of belly-crawling that he learned seemed like a small miracle because he was a child who disliked TummyTime and struggled to get mobile. Belly-crawling first started when my son made one big push with his big toe to get a toy that was just out of reach. After doing this for a week or so, he began moving a bit further. We noticed that it was much easier for him to do this on his right side and difficult on the left. Lenore taught us how to help him use his left side more. As she often said, "the goal is not symmetry, it's just more use on the less-used side". This was good to hear. It took the pressure off me to 'fix' something. It felt good just to give my son extra opportunities to work on the side that was more difficult and to feel I was possibly making things a little easier for him down the road. Lenore showed us the practices and encouraged us to find a regular time most days to work with what we had learned. Again, no pressure. Now, after several weeks, my son belly-crawls across the room when he is motivated by a toy or a mischievous errand.

A mother

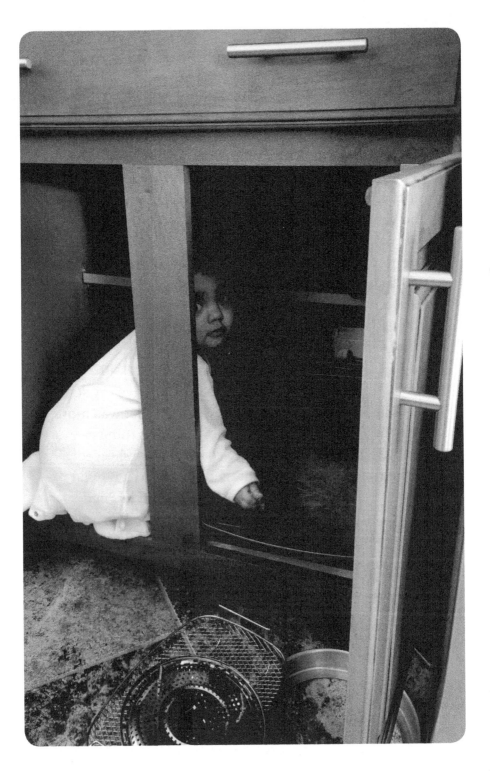

Ⓟractice:

Baby's Rest and Play in the Cupboards

One of the benefits of crawling for Baby is to be able to explore her home. It's really nice of you to allot a few cupboards, or some other space close to where you do most of your work in the kitchen, to let Baby play. Fill it with baby-safe yet 'real' stuff and let her do her thing there. Baby loves the cupboards in part because you do. She sees you opening and closing them and wants to do the same. And Baby loves the mystery of open and close. She may be hooked on this fascinating phenomenon, and apply it to various doors in your abode, for a long while.

As Baby plays in this safe place you have made for her, you can keep each other company while you tend to the kitchen and she increases her body awareness, her movement skills, and her sense of place in the home, the family, and her imagination.

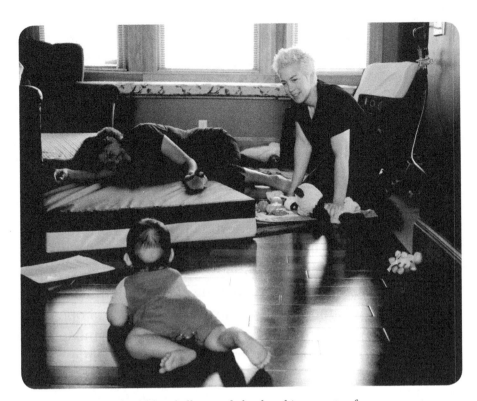

This seven-month-old boy belly-crawls back to his parents after exploring the next room.

Taking Care along the Way

Baby's earliest infancy was a time when she needed so much from you most of the time.

Now, she still needs you very much. However, she has become a Baby who no longer stays only where you place her. She can roll and belly-crawl on purpose. She can move to what she wants.

This new movement independence of Baby's may also feel bittersweet to you. It marks the end of your first chapter with Baby, the one of complete physical dependence.

In fact, Baby's secure feeling that you are there supports her movement away on her own adventures toward things of interest — and whatever she finds on the way.

It's joyful that Baby can move independently on the floor now. Especially if you make an area where she is safe to play and move and can see you from any spot in the area.

This changes the physical dynamics between you and Baby, but your emotional connection continues. You are still Baby's home base. This new stage of growing up involves periods of play when Baby moves away and comes back, again and again. She prefers that you stay where she left you and may become upset if you have moved when she sets out to belly-crawl back to you.

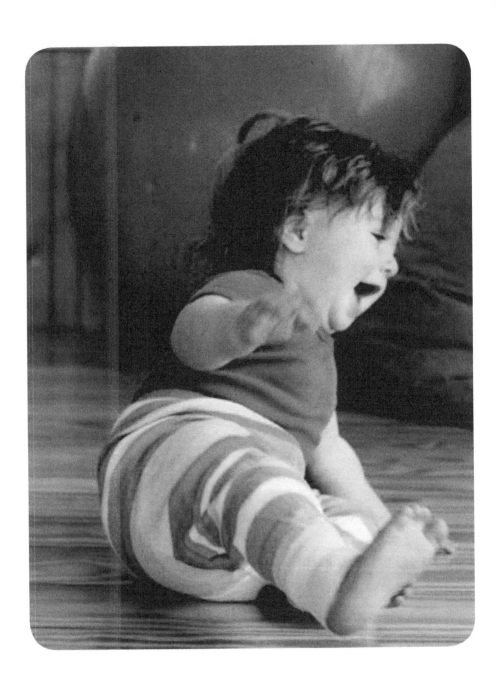

Belly-Crawling *Leads to:*

- *joyful, free body-play and independent movement at home.*
- *variations of leaning and pushing up to side-sitting.*
- *pulling up to hands-and-knees crawling.*
- *easier access to side-stepping once she learns to stand.*
- *beneficial connections between the sides of her brain, supporting language and learning.*

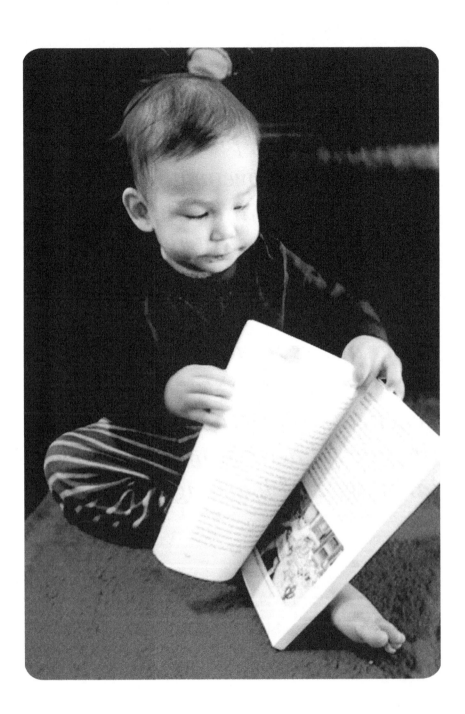

8. Learning To Sit Naturally

The way to natural sitting includes many variations of leaning. The next practices help you understand how to make leaning part of Baby's life. Sitting frees Baby's hands for fine motor play, encourages socializing, as well as stringing sounds together for "chatting." Sitting is the harvest of all the in-between strength-building that Baby has been doing.

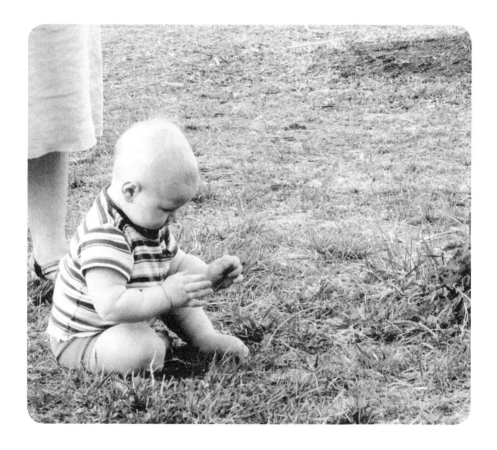

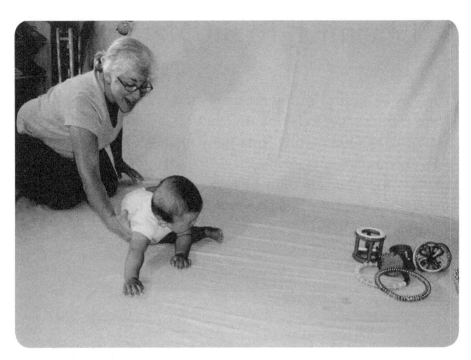

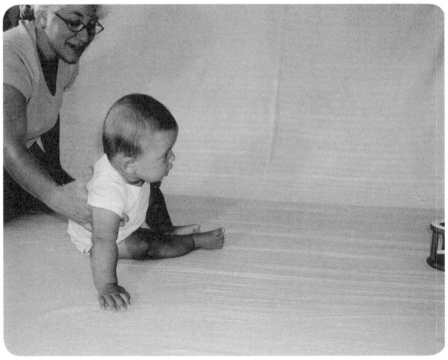

On the Way to Walking

(P)ractice

Side-Lying to Sitting

To move Baby from side-lying to sitting, you will actually *tip him up*. Place one hand over his ribs and under his arm. Lean his spine slightly forward so that he doesn't tighten his back as you tip his trunk up to sitting. With your other hand keep Baby's hip in contact with the floor so that his weight is primarily in his bottom, not on your arm.

Baby will gradually learn to do this on his own. He will practice self-supporting with his arm, his abs, his legs. He'll do lots of variations along the way to independent sitting—hopefully playfully and without too much unexpected falling! Usually after the first fall or two, Baby's brain and body learn how to prevent this falling from happening again. However, when tired, all of us are more prone to falling.

      When Lenore first introduced me to the practice of helping my baby move from lying down to sitting. I felt a little unsure as to where to put my hands. Nevertheless, we kept trying, and it got easier. After a few days it became second nature. After a few weeks, my Baby moves through these positions without any help.

Mother of a six-month-old

Tipping and Leaning

Parents often hold Baby upright in sitting.
It's equally important to hold Baby at a gentle
angle. Leaning, tipping, and *safe small falls* toward
his interest are essential to Baby's natural and
independent movement. Let Baby lean and tip when
you feel him reaching toward something. Give him
the chance to lean safely toward his interest when he
is in your arms, your lap, or on the floor. Tipping and
leaning engage the reflexes that are a part of every
gain in Natural Movement Development.

If you are new to lap-leaning, add some rhythmic
humming or singing. Please rock Baby, don't jiggle.

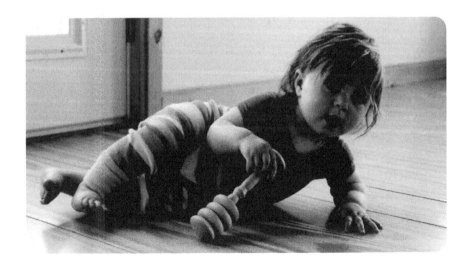

Sitting to Side-Leaning and Side-Lying

• If you are holding your baby in sitting and you are going to put him on the floor, lower him so that he lands on his side. Do this slowly with his neck slightly bent forward to avoid triggering his startle reflex as he goes down. If he startles, pick him up and wait until he settles to try again.

• In the earliest weeks, Baby is not able to extend his arm as he feels himself moving toward the floor. After that, each week he increases his activity in his arm on the floor side when he feels himself tipping. Each week as you lean him down, note how his arm on the lower side reaches out more and more toward the floor.

• Sometimes Baby tightens his waist and thrusts his legs as you lean him. In this case, slowly bring him back to upright sitting. Let him regroup, then gently tip his head and torso forward just slightly to ensure that his waist is bent forward as he goes down. This bend is essential for him to have because it engages the reflexes that support safe, independent movement in to, and out of, sitting.

• This is another time when Baby learns to use flexion. You and Baby may have reduced strong thrusting of the legs in recent weeks. Yet, when learning a new skill, particularly when changing levels, thrusting comes back to help Baby stay stable. Every time Baby leans to his side without falling back he reduces reflexive arching of his neck and thrusting of his legs. If he falls safely forward here, ideally with no pain, Baby how to move without falling from sitting to side-lying.

233

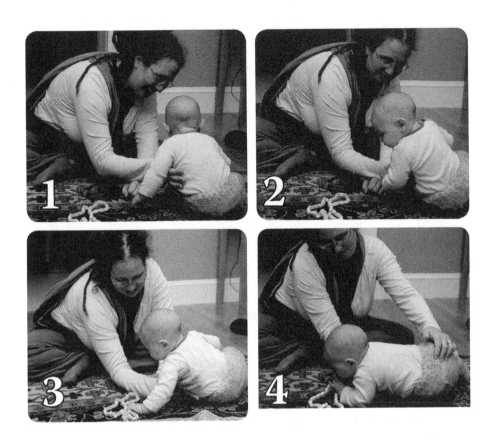

Move the Toy

When Baby wants to sit up to play with something, entice him by moving the toy. When he starts on his side or his belly and pushes up to sit, he moves a quarter-circle away from where he was. If possible, move the toy again to directly in front of him after he sits. Soon he'll be getting the toy himself.

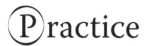ractice

Sitting to Side-Lying

In this photo sequence, Mom gives her six-month-old a light touch to help him lower himself to the floor without falling back. She keeps one hand under his ribs, ready to slide it away as soon as he regains his balance. This way her hand is not caught under Baby when he gets to the floor.

Mom doesn't do the movement for Baby. She observes what he is trying to do and helps him move through the spot where he is vulnerable to falling back. Each time they do this together, Baby becomes more able to do it independently. He won't need her help at all after a little more practice.

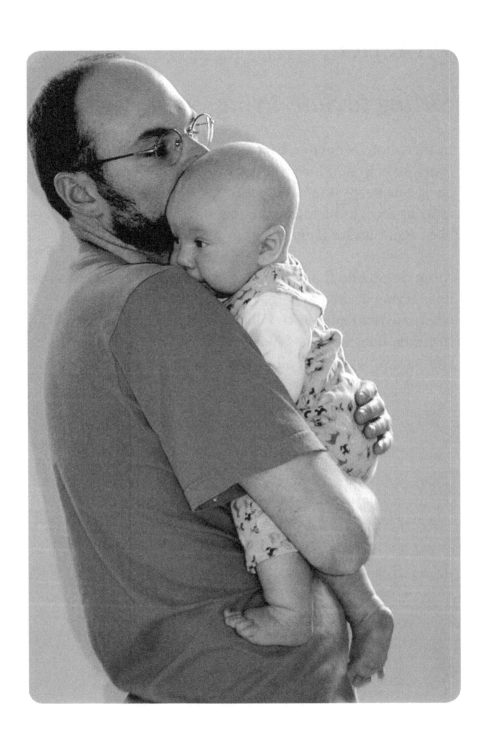

Natural Alternatives to Prop-Sitting

- Wearing Baby with fabric support under his whole bottom.
- Laying Baby on all four of his sides.
- Leaning Baby a bit to one side in your lap.
- Holding Baby under his bottom while he leans on your shoulder.
- Help Baby learn to move from side-lying to side-leaning to sitting, over many months.

Baby's efforts to move in and out of sitting typically coincide with his work on belly-crawling. In this phase Baby will sometimes surprise you by wanting to spend more time on his belly than his back. He also vocalizes more, and more loudly, on his belly!

Before Baby can sit independently, he will still spend plenty of time with his head and torso upright. When Baby wants to see a visitor, let him lean back against you when he is facing out, so he is supported while sitting and looking.

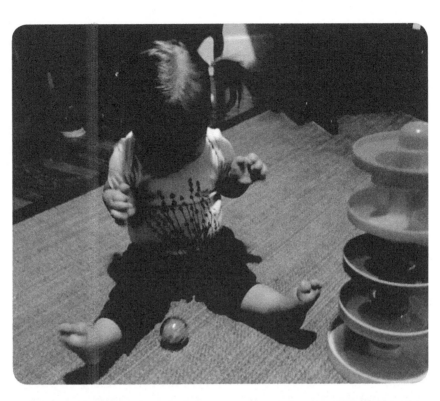

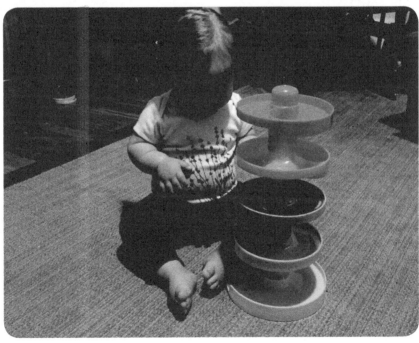

(P)ractice

Tucking the Toy on the Less Familiar Side in Sitting

The baby girl at left is excited to play with the orange ball. As part of her excitement she thrusts her legs. To help her decrease tight thrusting when sitting, and to help her to increase her core strength, gently bend one of her legs towards the other and slide a toy in front of that shin. Baby might pop her leg right out again. That's fine. This girl plays more easily over her right side. In the bottom left image, we see that Mom moved the tower in front of Baby's left leg to help her look and lean to her less familiar side.

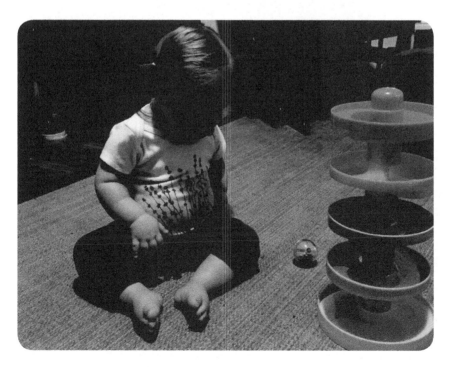

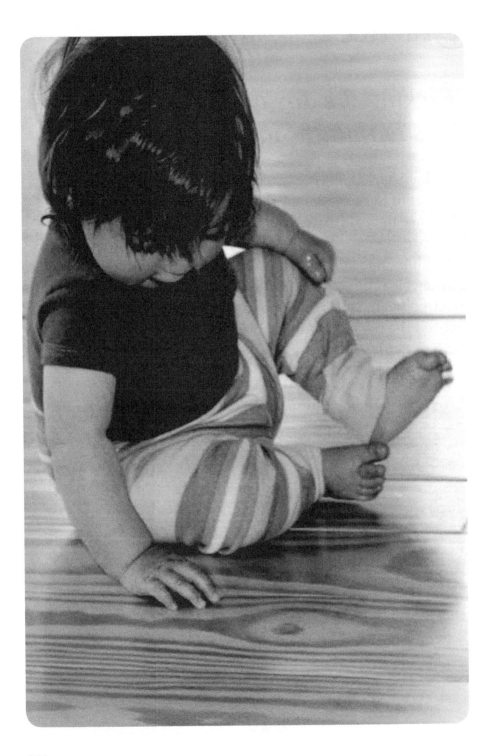

Sitting to Moving Freely

From comfortable sitting, Baby can bend one leg and tip forward. Over time, he tips all the way onto his arms and down to his tummy. As he gets stronger, he'll tip onto his hands-and-knees, then down to his tummy.

One day, while moving from sitting to hands-and-knees, he'll stay and rock there and reach out with his arm and take his first crawl step or two.

For days or weeks he'll move on hands-and-knees a little, dropping to his tummy when tired or the terrain is unstable, such as crawling over toys. Soon he'll mostly get about on all fours to play with something in his hands and mouth. He may still choose to be on his tummy or push back to sitting.

Baby has many movement choices now. He is happy to be moving about, and likely to be vocalizing more, and more loudly, to let you know about his discoveries!

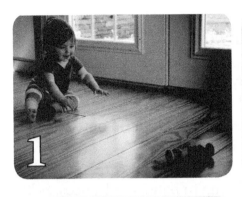

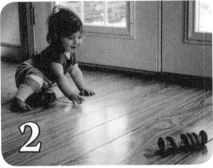

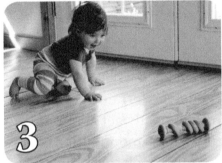

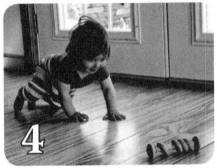

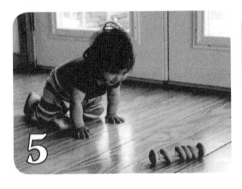

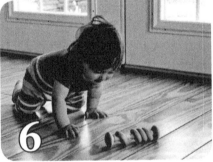

Go, Pause, Go

The busy baby hardly ever stops. When he does, it is usually to focus on something specific. Once he has explored that thing, off he goes again...all day long, with brief but frequent snacks on the way.

When Baby crawls to your lap, he doesn't need to be picked up as often as he used to. He comes in for contact, keeps his weight in his knees (even as he leans against you), and then, before you know it, he's done. He pivots on his knees, drops to hands-and-knees, and crawls away.

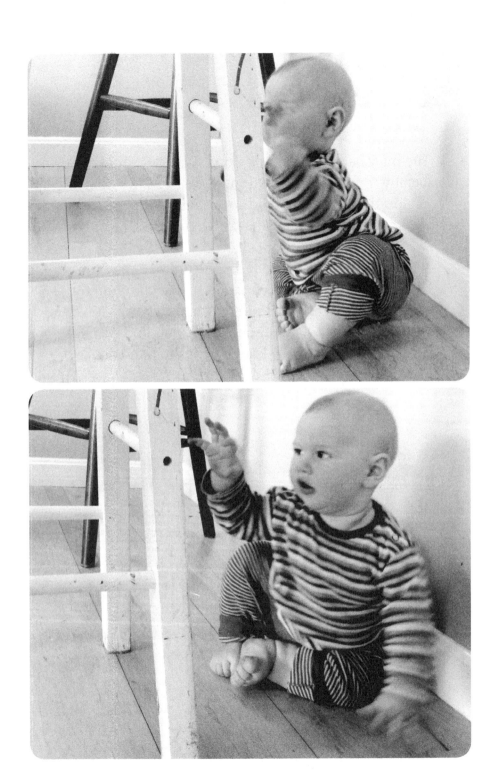

$\textstyle\bigodot$ractice

Tipping to Both Sides

From sitting, it is natural for Baby to be able to tip to his left or his right. If he is new to sitting, he will tip down to the floor and belly-crawl. His rhythm will be belly-crawl, sit, belly-crawl, sit.

Once he shifts from belly-crawling to hands-and-knees crawling, his rhythm will change. Now his rhythm will be hands-and-knees crawl, sit, hands-and-knees crawl, sit, and so on.

After hands-and-knees crawling, he will be interested in pulling himself up to standing. Now his rhythm will be hands-and-knees crawl, stand, hands-and-knees crawl, stand, etc. No longer just starting to get around, Baby is always getting all around!

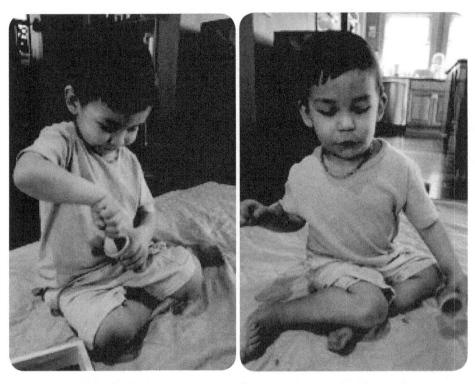

This two-and-a-half year-old was busy with his clay, then happily shifted his legs to his other side at our request, and continued his play.

Try It Yourself

Side-Sitting to Both Sides

Make some space on the floor and put out an object that elicits curiosity. Without thinking about it, sit down on the floor and lean toward the object. Pull it to you and sit up. Now, notice which side you chose.

Take the object and place it out at a forty-five degree angle on your less familiar side. Gently lean over and get it, bringing it toward you as you sit back up.

What did you feel?

Would you like to try it again?

This simple exercise of sitting to your less preferred side is a nice way to spend time with Baby, sharing some of what he is learning in your own way and showing embodied empathy.

Just as for Baby, there is no need to stay in the position if you are not comfortable. Just trying it is good for your body and mind.

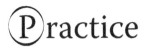ractice

Picking Up Baby from Sitting

Let Baby get ready by cueing him with the same words each time, such as "up." First, lean over and hold Baby by his waist. Gently lean him to one side. Next, swing Baby's shins behind him so that he shifts from sitting to kneeling. Both you and he will become accustomed to doing this. It's fine to tip him to the easier side when you need to get somewhere. Practice on the other side if you have an extra moment. Slide your forearm under his shins and pick Baby up from there.

Now you can get your other forearm under his bottom so that you are holding him in the usual way. Kneeling is an interim position you use so that he doesn't have to bear weight in his legs if he isn't ready to stand. And using this position you won't have to hang him by his armpits when you need to move him from one place to another.

This practice, like all of them, becomes easier for Baby and you after the first few times.

(P)ractice

From Your Arms to Side-Sitting

- Note which side baby leans over and which knee is up. It may not always be the same side, but it might.

- Place him down from your arms into the opposite side once or twice a day.

- Play or read in this position for a few minutes a day.

Short sessions, when he's allowed to move out of the position if he wants to, are best.

This practice is a simple, effective, and enduring tool to help Baby's use his less familiar side in daily life. You can create a routine of putting Baby down from your arms into his less familiar hip. It can be easy and lets you do so much for Baby with little effort. And it does not need to be done all the time, that is not the goal.

You may want to use a system to remember, because it can be confusing as to which is the familiar side. Something simple, such as a ring you wear or a freckle on one hand, to give you the friendly reminder of which side to place Baby.

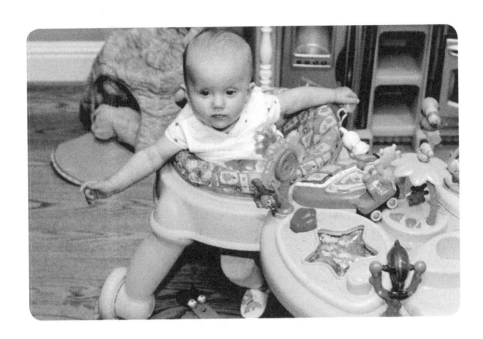

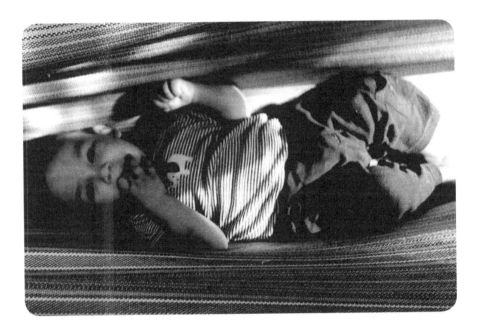

The girl at the top left is hanging by her crotch in a seat inside the walker. She spreads her arms out for balance. This walker makes Baby grow accustomed to leaning forward without falling. By moving in this way, she learns to fall without engaging the protective reflex responses in her arms. For some children, this has lasting physical and psychological impact.

The boy in the bottom photo is resting with his spine fully supported. He can sway in the hammock and look about, just as the girl above can move in the walker and look about.

A key difference in these two choices is that the girl is restricted in the walker, which allows her to move only by pulling herself along with her toes. The boy can move his whole body.

Alternatives to propping equipment include:

• Rocking bassinets.
• Infant swings.
• Inclined bouncing chairs.
• Simple buckets and baskets to help Baby keep busy in independent lying and sitting without being propped up.

If you use propping equipment at all, save it for stressed times when you need a safe, predictable place for Baby to be for a few minutes.

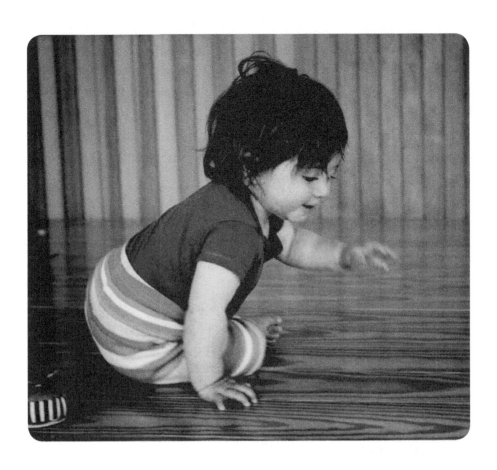

On the Way to Walking

Learning To Sit Naturally
Leads to:

- *a variety of movements, such as leaning into one hand and rocking on hands-and-knees.*
- *more fine motor skills.*
- *more utterances and stringing together of sounds.*
- *hands-and-knees crawling which leads to kneeling.*
- *busy, busy.*

Busy, Busy

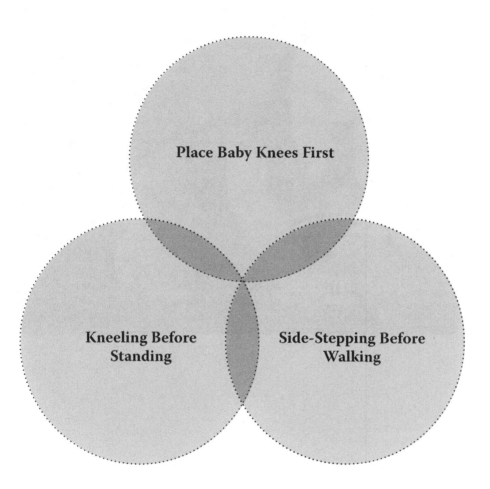

Place Baby Knees First

Kneeling Before
Standing

Side-Stepping Before
Walking

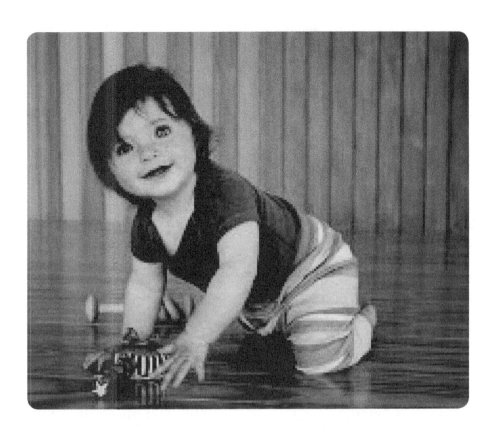

9. Hands-and-Knees Crawling

Crawling on hands-and-knees is the first time that Baby maintains her torso off the ground during movement. This is a big change for her, requiring more strength and coordination than belly-crawling.

Skillful belly-crawling, along with her growing curiosity, leads to hands-and-knees crawling. Now, when Baby reaches with one hand, her leg on the opposite side moves. This is her first hands-and-knees "step". These movements, sometimes referred to as *cross-crawling**, require and stimulate new areas in the middle of her brain and areas across her brain. All of this helps emotional, social, and cognitive development.

There is often a period when baby combines belly-crawling, hands-and-knees crawling, and pushing to sit. She's having fun feeling her body and figuring things out. Gradually she's becoming more skillful at hands-and-knees crawling, especially when she's mostly crawling before standing. She's becoming a fast, agile, *all-terrain baby**.

What's happening here?

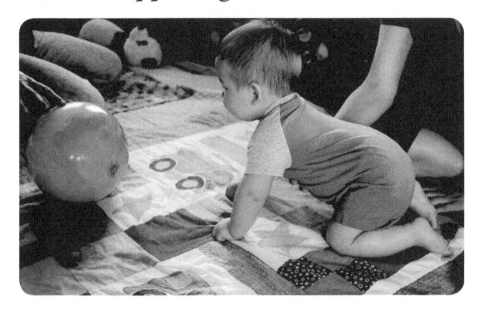

This seven-month-old boy and his parents are playing on the floor.
He is rocking on his hands-and-knees, a natural developmental
movement pattern, and talking to the ball.

Rocking on Hands-and-Knees

Some babies "pop up" to hands-and-knees from their bellies. This looks cute, and exciting. However, if Baby gets into the habit of popping up, she might lose the opportunity to belly-crawl. She will likely need to rock on hands-and-knees for days or weeks before she is strong enough to reach out with one hand and respond with the opposite knee, her first crawl step.

She may rock a lot and make a lot of sounds. Rocking on hands-and-knees feels good to Baby. It is both exciting and sometimes frustrating to be on her hands-and-knees and not be able to move through space.

Going from TummyTime to rocking on hands-and-knees, to crawling forward happens. It's just easier for Baby if she finds belly locomotion before she gets up on her knees.

At ten months and up, a toddler-sized slide will be a great toy for her. Working on climbing up the slide, with your help under each foot, will give her another chance to move with the belly crawling pattern. The angle and challenge of the slide tends to bring this out.

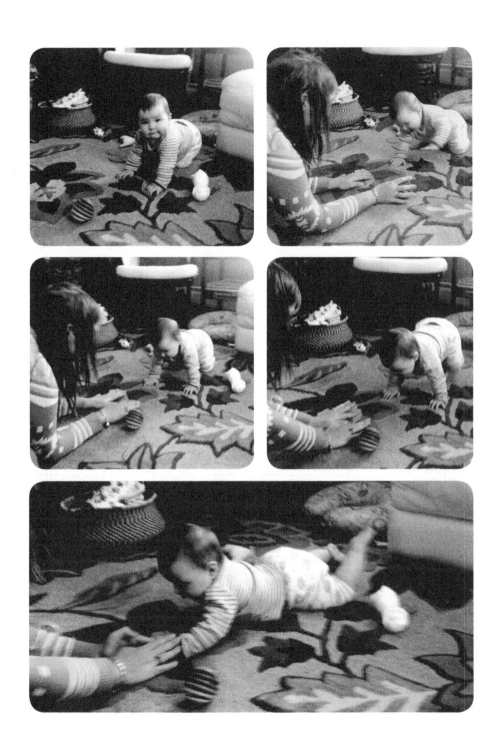

Lots of Skills and Positions Are Going On

Baby can do so much now:

• She belly-crawls.

• She reaches and grabs and holds on.

• She rocks on her hands-and-knees.

• She does the airplane when on her tummy.

• She three-point-crawls, lifting one hand off the floor.

• She bear-stands with her bottom up and her hands and feet on the floor.

What a girl! She barely has time to nurse before she's off to the next thing!

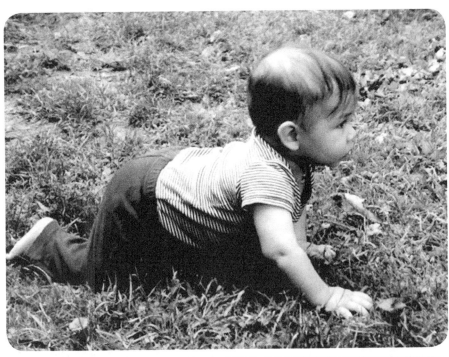

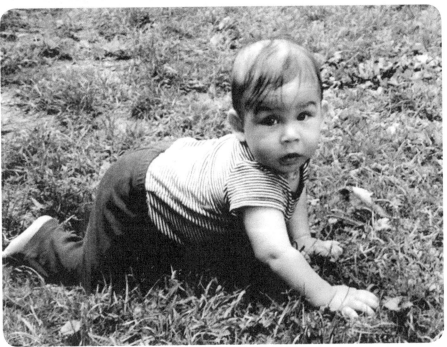

Hands-and-Knees Get Going

After rocking on her hands-and-knees, Baby starts to move. Uh oh, here she comes! She reaches out with one hand and her opposite knee follows. Then she reaches out with the other hand and the other opposite knee follows.

At first she'll take a crawl-step or two, and then drop down to her belly again. She may not do it again for a day or two, then her crawling sequences might get a little longer. Over days and weeks Baby becomes a speedy crawler. She will be an expert who will not stop for objects in the way—she will crawl right over them. A parent once called this familiarity and confidence in hands-and-knees crawling the *all-terrain-baby**, and the term has stuck.

The sequence of interest and attention in hands-and-knees crawling is:

- Interest in something and the desire to move toward it.
- From hands-and-knees a reach forward of one hand.
- Followed by a step of the opposite knee.
- Followed by a reach of the other hand.
- Followed by a step of the opposite knee.
- Able to sit back from crawling while holding an object.

Later, walking upright, Baby uses a similar sequence of movements while her weight is over her legs and feet.

Sitting Back from Hands-and-Knees Crawling

When Baby crawls on hands-and-knees, she sits back to one side after she reaches her destination.

The side Baby sits back to is not going to be a surprise. As we have been discussing all along, it will be the same side she leaned on in her lower, younger movements.

Once Baby can sit back to both sides, she is ready to sit back in her middle, which is kneeling. This is the hardest of these three choices. By sitting back left and right, she builds strength to sit back into kneeling.

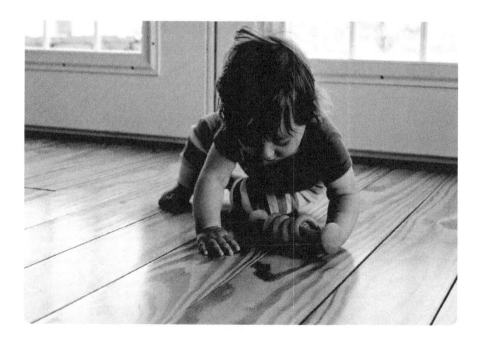

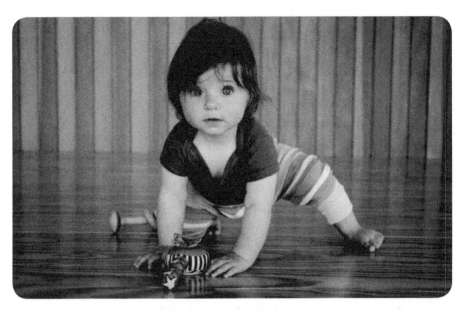

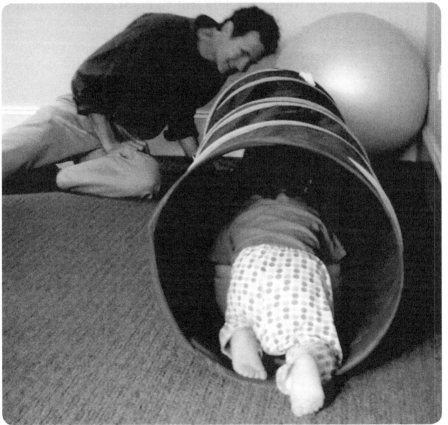

Crawling with One Knee Up

Sometimes Baby crawls on two hands and one knee with the other knee up and the foot on the floor. The knee touching the floor is on the weight-bearing side (this is called *crab-crawling**). This will be the same side that she found easier to lie on, to roll toward, and to sit back on from crawling.

When you see Baby crawling with one knee up, refer to the kneeling practices in this book. With these practices many infants who are crawling with one knee up learn to crawl with both knees down. This increases Baby's comfort, safety, and her speed, which she likes. It also helps her to build more symmetrical strength in the muscles of her trunk for the long term health of her spine, lower back, and knees.

The aim is to provide Baby with opportunities to crawl with her weight on both knees, at least sometimes. The goal is not to eliminate three-point crawling. It is to increase confidence and safety in hands-and-knees crawling.

If you use the practices in this book, Baby may still crawl with one knee up. This is not because you, or Baby, or the practices, are lacking. It is natural for Baby—and all of us—to lean to the more familiar side while she coordinates her new movements.

Baby may crab-crawl for a little while, then begin, with a little incentive from you, to crawl with both knees down. And sometimes, for reasons you can or can't guess, you might see her knee up again for a period.

ⓅPractice

Helping Baby To Hands-and-Knees Crawl with Both Knees Down

Be sure Baby is happily playing when you begin. Use toys that roll, make sounds, and engage her. When possible, invite siblings to play nearby. Baby's engagement in play is essential.

First, join Baby on the floor and play. Try crawling on your hands-and-knees while you play. Now gently try crawling with one of your knees up, like Baby does. Notice how this feels. Sit back and rest.

Observe Baby and note which of her knees does not touch the floor.

Crawl behind her and bring her knee to the floor as she moves. Place one hand gently on Baby's lifted knee and connect with her. Now, use that hand to move her lifted shin to the floor. Once her shin is on the floor, place your hand over the back of that calf to help keep her shin on the floor.

Additionally, when you are putting Baby down from your arms, place her onto the hip and knee that she does not usually put on the floor. Once she is on the floor, remove your hands. She may immediately switch back to her other side. It is valuable for her brain and body to experience bearing weight on her less familiar side, even briefly.

As soon as Baby rests into both knees, remove your hands. Her knee may pop right back up, or it may not. If it does, it is not because she doesn't want to "cooperate." Her knee pops up because of her connective tissue impression made during her time *in utero*.

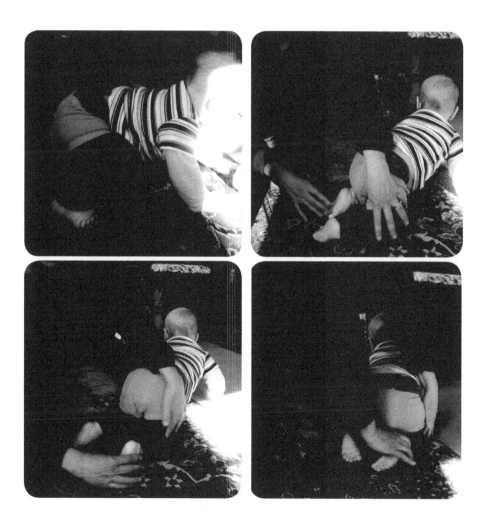

A Bit on Talking

Baby makes sounds from the first day. Initially her sounds are exclusively for survival. These sounds come from low in her brain and she doesn't choose whether or not to make them. While crying is first, Baby soon makes other sounds— inadvertently, and then intentionally.

As Baby's attention moves outward from her early InnerTime, she will be making sounds and hearing herself. If she discovers how to make a raspberry, she might do raspberries for weeks or months!

I notice babies start making sounds that are either mostly vowels or mostly consonants. They do both; yet, you will likely notice Baby doing more of one or the other. For example, she might make sounds that such as "aahh" and "ohh". Or, she might more often say "ma" or "ba" or "da." Once Baby finds a sound, she usually sticks to it. Baby will have an intentional first sound or two that she uses to greet, to name things, and to chat with visitors.

Imitate Baby from the beginning. Its fun, informative, and helps Baby learn to talk.

Baby's comprehension of speech is ahead of her ability to talk for a long time. She understands more than you may think, and more so with each passing week. Speak simply in your normal tone with Baby. Watch and listen carefully for her response, which she makes with her whole body, not only with sounds and words.

From Your Arms to Her Hands-and-Knees

Once Baby can crawl, you can put her down to her hands-and-knees from your arms. Hold her by her waist, letting her arms reach out. Lower her into her hands, then her knees. Off she goes!

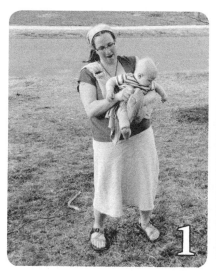

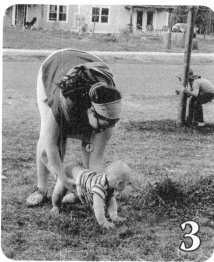

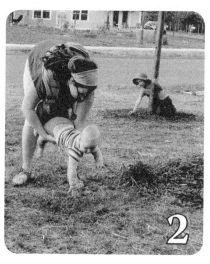

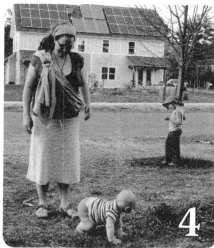

“ My son is currently practicing many of the pieces of hands-and-knees crawling. His main means of locomotion is belly-crawling, but he will often pause in other positions during his play. He is confident sitting while he plays, but if a toy rolls away from him, he will move forward onto his hands-and-knees. Then he might rock on hands-and-knees for a little while before releasing down to his belly and belly-crawling forward to get the toy.

He loves to climb in and out of my lap. When I sit and play with him on the floor, he uses my body as a jungle gym. He will pull up onto my leg and pivot to one side or the other and into a sitting position. Then he might pivot back to me and into a kneeling position. He does this over and over again and seems to be practicing for when he is confident enough to try it all on his own. ”

A Mother

Crawling before Standing

Baby's brain and body are designed to move forward on hands-and-knees before standing up and side-stepping or forward-walking. While many babies skip this stage and manage just fine with their brains and bodies, others benefit greatly from this fundamental skill set.

Crawling on hands-and-knees has been shown to help language development, motor coordination, even math and music skills.

After learning to crawl and kneel, Baby readily plants one foot or the other to push up to stand.

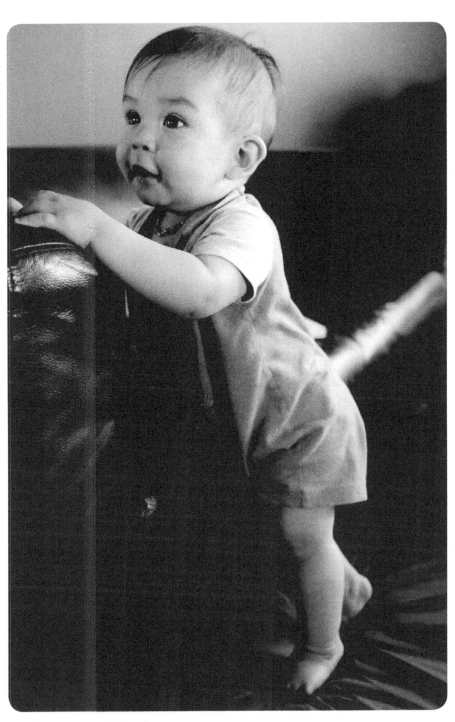

Pulling up to early standing.

Early Standing

This practice maximizes the developmental opportunities that belly-crawling and hands-and-knees-crawling provide Baby before standing. Even without propping, Baby can figure out how to pull up to standing before she has learned how to crawl on hands-and-knees. This is especially the case when Baby has strong thrusting of her legs, then she can tip from sitting, and pull herself up by rolling right over the tops of her toes. This premature standing is cute, yet it is not an indication of early prowess. With your help, Baby will soon enough be crawling, and then she'll be ready to push to standing using her whole brain and body.

It can feel good to Baby to encourage her to stand. It affords her a better view than previously and typically gets an excited response from grown-ups.

There is nothing wrong with early standing. However, parents don't know that, with a little assistance, Baby can learn how to find her way back down from standing. This is important because, if she only stands, she will do more and more leg thrusting, and could lose the opportunity to learn to crawl, and with it the flexibility of body and brain that crawling provides.

If Baby thrusts her legs strongly early on, she will likely stand early. When Baby thrusts often, it's easy to get in the habit of standing her, because her legs lock in this position. However, with knowledge that belly-crawling, kneeling, and crawling on hands-and-knees are essential skills prior to Baby's standing, we can cultivate them. Parents want Baby to experience these movements once they understand their essential value and the ease of including them in daily play.

ⓟractice

Getting Down from Early Standing

To help Baby down from early standing, be sure to connect with her first. Put your hands on her waist, with something of interest on the ground, and help her bend at her waist as she lowers her behind to the floor. This is sometimes a small fall. Baby can learn to do this in a controlled, intentional way. She'll learn to drop down from standing with ease. First, she will likely need a little help bending her waist now that she is standing.

Early standing indicates that Baby is good at thrusting her legs while not as comfortable bending them.

When you help her learn to drop down from her first early standing, she won't have to cry for help or be stuck standing.

Many Babies learn to drop back to their knees after discovering standing, and then go on to be adept hands-and-knees crawlers. After crawling Baby begins again to stand and side-step. Now Baby's reflexes and muscles on the front and back of her body support her to move up and down safely and independently.

“ My son also loves to "pop up" to standing. I can see by the way that he balances himself that he is not really ready to stand. When he pops up to standing, I help him to practice ways to get back down to the floor where he is more confident in movement. Lenore showed him how to "plop" himself back down to sitting. Now my son drops his bottom and sits back with a plop. After practicing this a few times, it became easy, and he really liked it. I know this is a good safety skill for him to have once he starts walking. ”

A Father

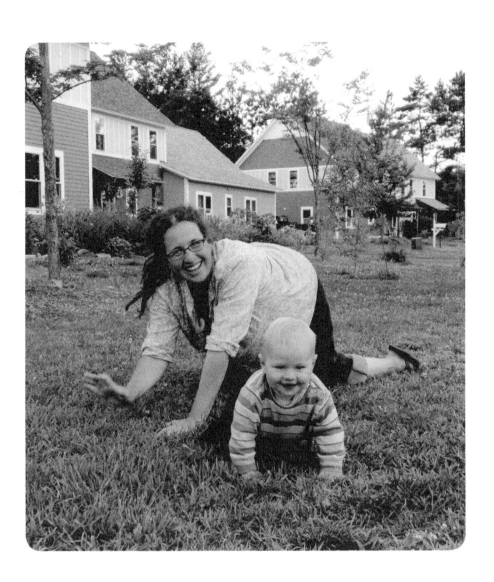

Try It Yourself

- Wear knee pads if you need them, or tie a scarf around each knee before you start.
- Crawl! Let Baby show you how. Let him see you crawling!
- Don't think about how you crawl. Keep your attention focused on him and the things around you instead of on what you are doing with your body.
- Imitate the sounds he's making as he crawls; let yourself play with sound.
- Rest when you want to.
- Later, for a moment, crawl more slowly, with attention. Notice which limb you usually start with. Sit back from crawling. Are you over your left hip, right hip, kneeling, or something else altogether? Your own developmental movement is still with you, there for the exploring.

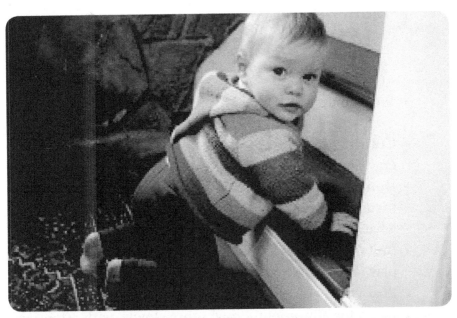

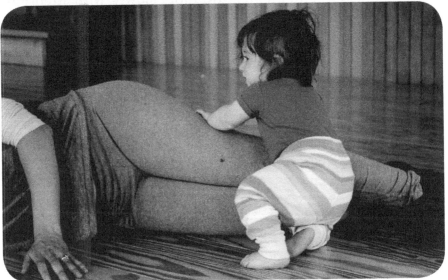

Hands-and-Knees Crawling
Leads to:

- *moving easily to one's interest.*
- *dropping back into side-sitting from hands-and-knees.*
- *dropping back into kneeling from hands-and-knees.*
- *pulling to stand.*
- *climbing.*
- *going up and down stairs.*
- *more socializing.*
- *playing catch.*
- *playing peek-a-boo.*
- *for some, a change in sleep patterns.*

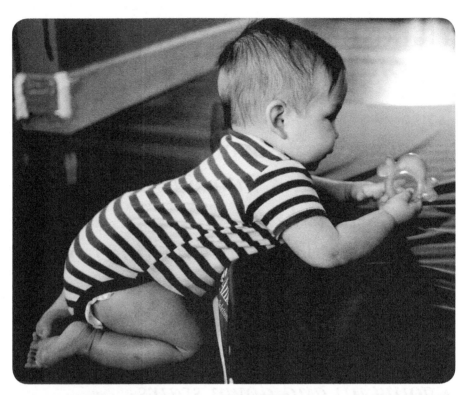

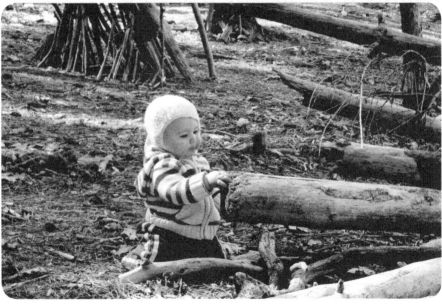

10. Kneeling, Knee-Standing, and Knee-Walking

Kneeling

Kneeling is nature's insurance policy. It is another chance to help Baby feel oriented and to strengthen his body in essential ways.

First, he will move out of all fours to sit back over one leg in side-sitting. After some weeks of sitting back to the left or the right, he'll be ready for some help to learn to sit directly back over his heels, which strengthens both sides of his body.

Kneeling, and all movement variations from there, are natural and helpful to Baby. They provide a strong base out of which hands-and-knees crawling, standing and walking grow. It is ideal for Baby's brain and body if he learns to rock on hands-and-knees before kneeling, and kneel before standing, side-stepping, and walking.

Babies can miss the opportunity to move through these valuable positions when caregivers are not aware of their importance and focus solely on Baby's sitting and standing. However, even if Baby has already done lots of early standing, kneeling can be learned, if taught gently and playfully.

Try It Yourself

Kneeling Strengthens the Trunk

Since we don't know how Baby feels while taking these positions and doing these movements, it is helpful to try them yourself.
Can you kneel?

Some people's knees or ankles will not tolerate full kneeling. How about trying knee-standing? It is a bit easier on the knees.

From there, try knee-walking. You will notice that you need to use muscles on the front of your body to protect your lower back when knee-walking.

Kneeling can rest the body and the spirit; a place and perspective between sitting, and standing. *(Use knee pads if you like.)*

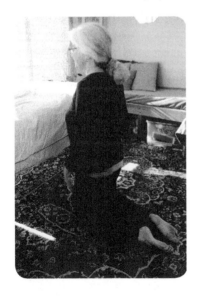

(P)ractice

Kneel Play

Kneeling play is beneficial for Baby and can easily be part
of everyday life. Use sturdy objects at his kneeling height.
A box with a blanket in it for weight, or a stool, supports
this essential natural position. This stimulates the
development of Baby's core strength in preparation for
standing later on (not too long from now).

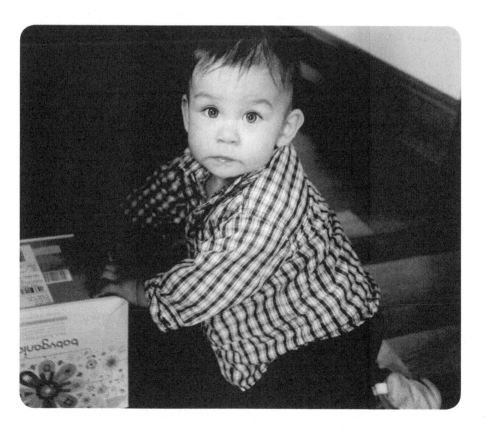

ⓅPractice

Helping Baby Sit Back into Kneeling

Sitting back directly over his heels from crawling is a natural position, yet it is one that Baby needs help finding. Kneeling helps Baby's trunk grow stronger to prepare for standing. Over time, Baby will kneel independently, building his base for his next budding movements.

When crawling on his hands-and-knees, he drops back to side-sitting when he is ready to sit down. Like all the other movements, he will use one side more than the other. Once you help him learn to sit back to both sides, then he is ready to learn to sit back into kneeling.

With this help, Baby learns to kneel back from his hands-and-knees without falling backward. Once you help him find this he will enjoy kneeling during play. Provide a box or table at just the right height for him to do this.

First, set up play situations that help him sit back to his less-used side. Observe which side Baby sits back into from his hands-and-knees, so you can be ready to help him sit back to his less familiar side.

If he has already started going down to the familiar side, you have missed your chance this time; wait for your chance the next time you anticipate he is about to sit back.

As you move him back, move the object of interest to within Baby's reach as he sits back. At first keep your hand behind his back. If he is not ready he will slip to side-sitting.

It may feel awkward at first, until Baby's reflex for kneeling is engaged. Keep it playful, brief, and not too goal-oriented. Having the experience is more essential than staying there.

Place your hands on either side of his waist and pull his tail directly toward his heels. As soon as he starts to sit back, remove your hands. If he is wobbly, keep your hands near without touching.

Each time he grows a little, he might need a little help again with kneeling back. Then, he will be doing it freely on his own when he wants to.

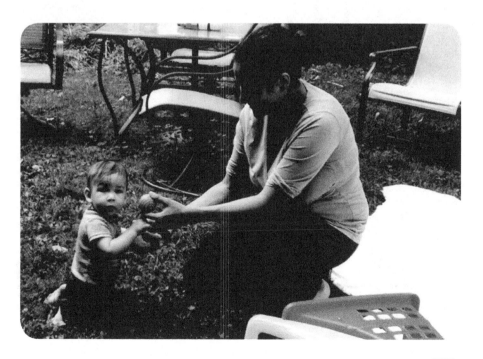

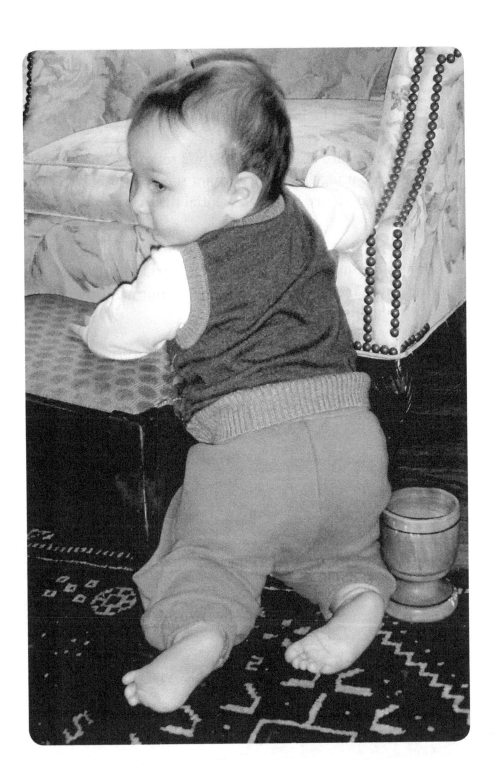

Ankle Twists Are Deep

Our two ankles are not perfectly straight and they are not identical. The connective tissue in the ankles is strongly imprinted from our position *in utero.* Baby may have one or both ankles noticeably turned or twisted.

Sitting over his heels, Baby stimulates reflexes by bearing weight into his ankles. These reflexes support alignment of the ankle, knee, and hip.

From kneeling, Baby plants his foot on his familiar side to push up. With your help, he will occasionally plant his less familiar foot to stand up. This, along with learning to kneel back over both his heels, naturally aids alignment of Baby's ankles over time.

Many of us feel tight in our ankles and feel discomfort in our ankles when on our hands-and-knees.

When helping Baby, and when trying it yourself, approach gently and kindly. Provide touch to kindly position the ankle more straight. It doesn't need to be perfect and it doesn't need to stay where you place it. We help Baby feel a new position, ideally without physical or personal upset. His ankle shifts from more stiff to more flexible, even if he moves it back into the twist after your touch.

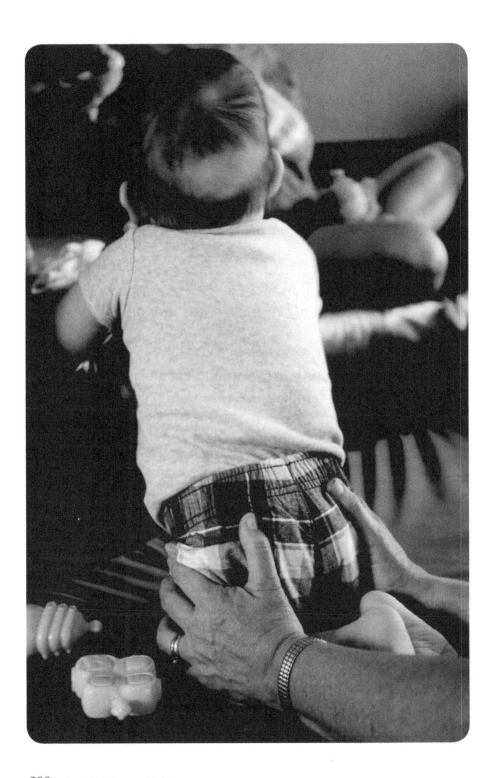

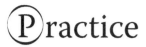

Practice

Narrowing Baby's Base in Kneeling

Baby knees may tend to slide wide apart while he is kneeling in play. Like other natural movements that need attention to grow best, Baby benefits when you narrow his base of support while he is kneeling. This means helping Baby feel his legs directly under his pelvis to help him strengthen his trunk. Trunk strength helps Baby's balance on his way to walking and beyond. Narrowing Baby's base, whether with your hands, as at left, or by sitting behind him with your thighs on either side of his, is a more upright, bigger-Baby version of Baby Ball.

1. Sit next to Baby on the floor. Start by connecting with play and touch. Be sure Baby is busy with something interesting when you practice. Proceed slowly so as not to cause him to fall forward without time to put out his arms.

2. Narrow Baby's base in small increments by tipping his pelvis slightly to one side, tucking his opposite lower leg under his thigh, next tipping him gently to the other side and tucking that lower leg on that side. Continue little tips and tucks, back and forth, to bring his calves under his thighs, moving his upper body as little as needed.

3. Try once or twice a day during play, for a week or two, until Baby kneels independently. As he grows, you'll see his base widen again. After a growth spurt, return to narrowing Baby's base in play.

As you remove your hands from Baby's legs, briefly stroke his ankle and slightly move his foot more in line with his shin.

Narrowing Baby's Base Is Good for Him

Welcome the opportunity to narrow Baby's base when he is busy playing with small things, then remove your hands quickly. Some children will stay and some will slip back to a wider base after a few seconds. Staying in the position is not as important for Baby as having moments there while playing. Baby might enjoy having you kneel behind him, helping him to keep his base narrow with your body.

His legs might slide wide again; however, even brief stays provide beneficial stimulation of reflexes which strengthen Baby's trunk for balance and flexibility.

" I like it when my mom brings my knees together when I am kneeling and playing. The first few times it felt a little scary. I was afraid I was going to fall. Now I can feel that I am strong enough not to fall. I don't like it when my knees start to slide apart while I am playing. It is uncomfortable and I don't feel as strong. I feel good when she tucks my legs under me. After all, I will need my legs under me when I want to take off crawling. Thanks, mom! "

Speaking for Baby

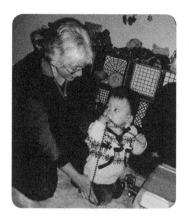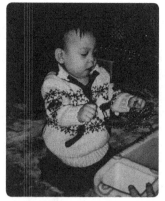

Lenore kneels around this boy as she helps narrow his base. She backs off as he continues to play. The kneeling table is essential when narrowing Baby's base.

(P)ractice

Helping Baby Shift from Kneeling to Hands-and-Knees

Baby may get comfortable kneeling and then need a little help for a little while to learn to shift to his hands-and-knees.

To help Baby move comfortably from kneeling to hands-and-knees, put a toy in front of him and sit behind him with your legs outside of his legs. Place one hand on his front. When you feel Baby leaning forward to the toy, use your body and your hand to help him tip until one or both of his arms come out. He can choose to stay on his hands-and-knees, or sit back into kneeling, no urgency. This practice can progress readily from a little scary, to familiar, to a fun and natural part of movement.

What's happening here?

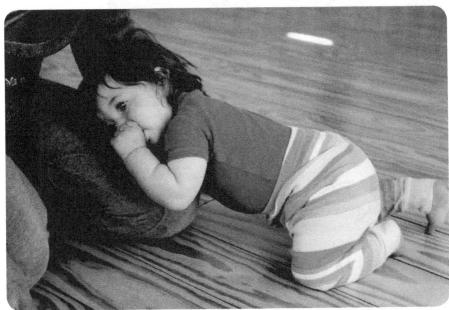

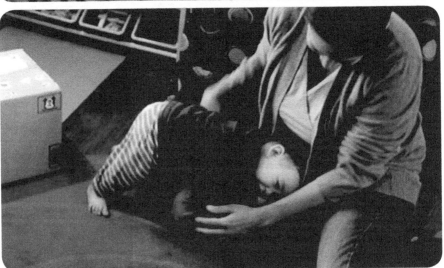

These parent-child teams show us loving lap pauses in the life of "go, pause, go."

ⓅPractice:

Your Lap Is Important

Once your Baby can crawl toward and away from you, he may, sometimes, come by just for a brief visit. He may stay on his hands-and-knees or he may pull himself up to kneeling to get closer to your face. Other times, he may want to climb on, or over, you. He doesn't need assistance unless he cries for it.

When your baby was smaller, it was automatic to pick him up. Now it's a learning step for you, the parent, to let him come by for a visit, connect, not pick him up, and let him move along as he wants to.

Parents may not realize what a valuable resource their own laps are for Baby's play. This is a great place for Baby to learn to move in many ways. Particularly, he can practice kneeling. He can do essential strength building in his arms when he intentionally tips forward from your lap to the floor. He lands on his hands and learns to safely support himself with his arms without falling, or with safe small falls. Variations of lap play usually go on for months when allowed.

Lap play is not a fit for everybody. Please do not feel you must do it if you are not comfortable. A few big pillows, balls, or bolsters on the floor work well for Baby to crawl on and kneel at while you're nearby.

Knee-Standing

Soon Baby can stand on his knees. We cultivate knee-standing with engaging play. We refrain from picking up Baby automatically, as we do when he is younger. Then, we always picked him up. Now, he connects with you while kneeling, keeping his weight on the floor, without needing you to pick him up.

Baby may play while crawling, kneeling, and sitting for many weeks. Some babies will knee-step, taking a step or two on their knees. This occurs when a supporting object that he is leaning on moves or an enticing object is out of reach. If he becomes aware over time that the supporting object can move and that he is the one that can move it, then he might use it to move around. This is knee-walking.

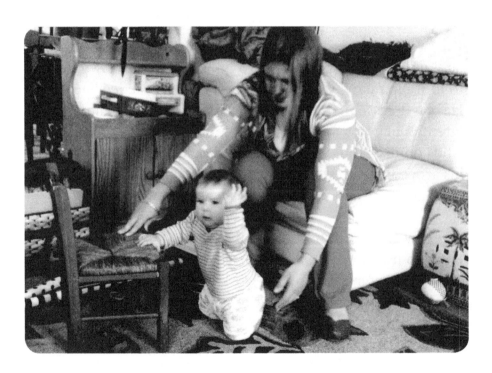

Reflexes Have Many Natural Chances To Bloom

Kneeling, knee-standing, and knee-walking are all parts of nature's insurance policy for Baby's development. They provide new opportunities for him to strengthen his trunk with flexor muscles, whether he had TummyTime, or belly-crawled, or not. If Baby didn't spend much time on his tummy in his earliest months, kneeling is a new opportunity for him to build essential flexion strength on the front of his body. This can help him bend his legs with more ease, an important skill when he is growing and doing a lot of strong thrusting of his legs. Further, kneeling makes Baby's abs stronger, which we all know is important. This strength keeps Baby more stable—and more able to fall without injury—and therefore, safer in all that he does.

Bear-Standing and Bear-Walking

Once Baby can rock on all fours, he sometimes finds a way to push with his arms and legs and his bottom goes up. He sometimes even moves in this position. Bottom up and head down with his weight in his hands and feet is called *bear-standing**.

If Baby steps while in this position it is called *bear-walking**. This is fun for Baby, but if he keeps his bottom in the air and can't bring his knees to the floor, he'll need a little help from you to learn to crawl on his hands-and-knees.

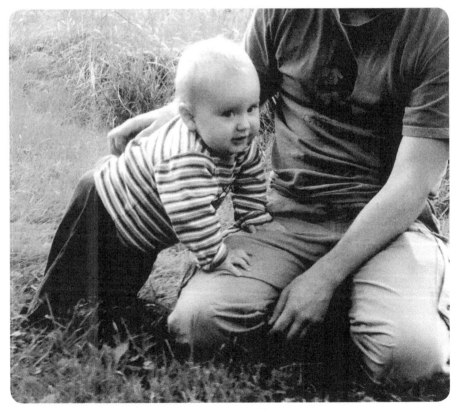

Bear-standing on Dad's thigh.

Ⓟractice

Bear-Walking to Hands-and-Knees Crawling

Find something enticing that you and Baby can play with on the floor. As he starts to move toward it help him bring one of his knees, and then the other, down to the ground as he moves. Often Baby is busy and doesn't want you to bother him while he plays. Therefore, bring his knees down for one or two steps and then quickly remove your hands.

Try brief moments of practice at least a couple of times a day for a few weeks. By then Baby may be used to crawling on hands-and-knees, or he may still need more time, and a little more of your help, to learn this.

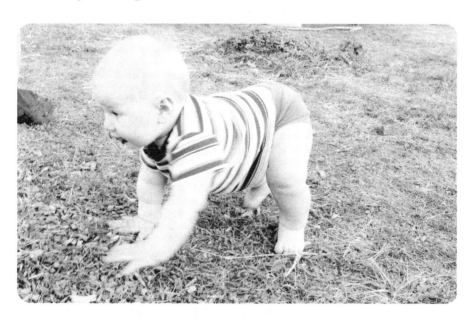

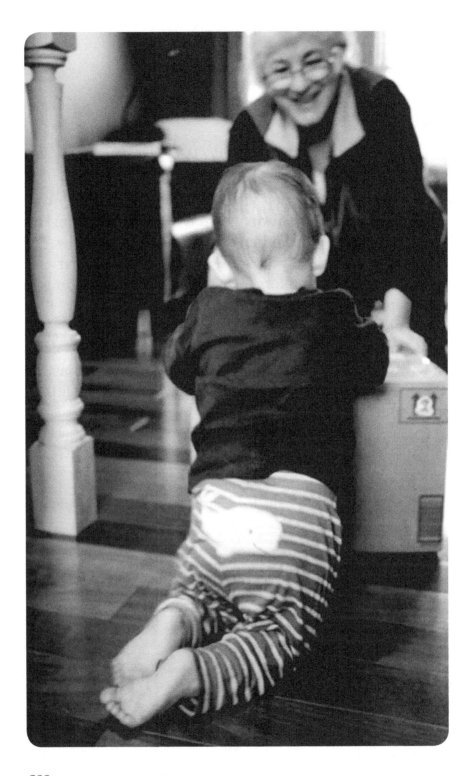

On the Way to Walking

Knee-Walking

*Knee-walking** is a natural and advantageous movement pattern. Babies don't generally do it because people don't know it is there to cultivate. Once your Baby can crawl on hands-and-knees, and after you have taught him to sit back into kneeling from hands-and-knees, you can entice him to take some knee-steps. The best way, as usual, is if you get down and do it yourself so that Baby can see what it is all about. Often Baby learns just because he saw you doing it.

If he can kneel independently, you can kneel behind him and help him take a few knee-steps. Tip and lift his leg as you tip and lift your own leg (just as you would do if he were standing on your feet and you were walking).

Knee-walking gives Baby a way to get around, helps make him stronger, and is another way he gets ready for safe standing. For babies who are developing slowly, and for those who may have low tone, it is actually better to knee-walk until Baby's natural impulse to stand occurs, based on his own strength.

Like all the prior movement patterns, they are not just good for Baby, they are fun too. Knee-walking continues to be a part of children's play at times, even when they can run, jump, and skip. Try it yourself. You will find that knee-walking requires your trunk strength. It's a bit like crawling upright. Do it on a carpet so your knees are protected and you can have fun.

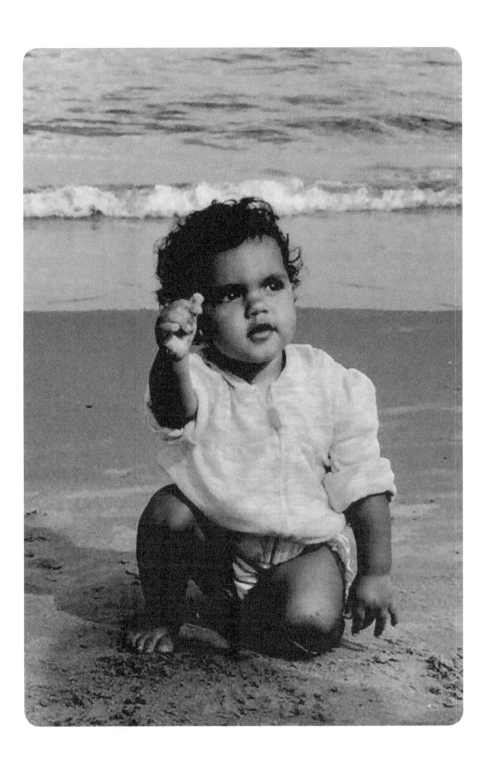

Half-Kneel-Sitting

This position is between kneeling and knee-standing!
It is a wonderful position on the way to kneeling and
standing and remains a part of movement play as children
grow. Baby is partly drawn to sit and is also ready to get back
on the move.

This is a position we use throughout life. Even when
we are sitting, we sometimes bring one knee up and
we are half-kneel-standing on the chair.

This reminds you to participate in your baby's fascination
with the world with your body, as well as your mind.
Don't forget to do it yourself—when your child is
half-kneel-standing to show you something. Look at
it in the same position as Baby.

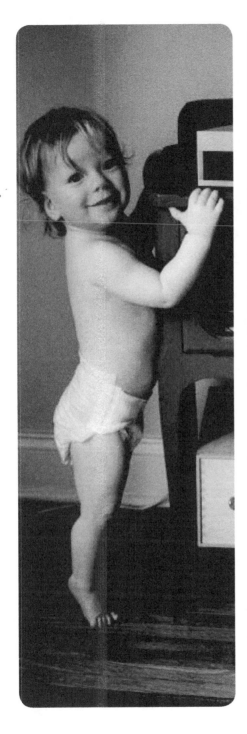
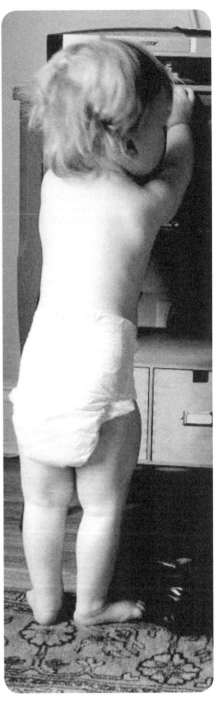

Kneeling, Knee-Standing, and Knee-Walking *Lead to:*

- *half-kneel-standing.*
- *standing.*
- *side-stepping.*
- *climbing people, furniture, and stairs.*
- *long-term low-back strength.*

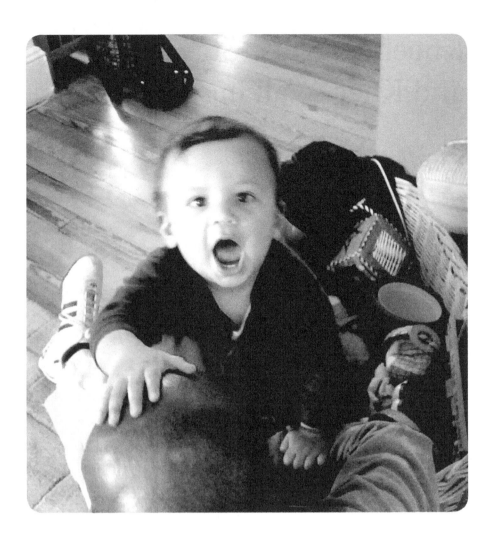

On the Way to Walking

11. Standing, Side-Stepping, Climbing, and Walking

Every Baby has a deep urge to get to stand.

Baby wants to see what everyone else can see. Things out of reach become interesting. Especially when she wants to reach them and can't!

Sometimes Baby pulls up to standing and is not aware of how she got there, although she may have been trying to pull up for some time.

Other times, Baby delights in standing. Then she cries because she can't get down. If Baby is not urged to walk, her natural rhythm in this period will likely be crawl, stand, crawl, stand. Then stand, side-step, stand. She does this until she is strong enough that she will spontaneously forward-step or walk. Even then, she may walk, side-step, walk until she gets stronger and will likely still drop to hands-and-knees when traversing irregular surfaces (such as a toy-strewn floor).

Ready For Standing:
Planting the Foot to Stand

When Baby is ready for standing, she plants the sole of her foot on the ground and pushes down into it as she also pulls herself up with her arms.

This new set of movement skills that work together take time to become coordinated, and Baby is going to do some interesting movement variations on the way. Take time to enjoy watching her figure it out.

When Baby attempts to stand, we will see her get ready by shifting her weight in her usual way, and lifting the other leg to plant that foot. This is a new, more vertical version of her familiar tendencies. In belly-crawling, Baby found it easier to lean over one side of her pelvis and bend her leg on the other side. This ease reappears as she changes levels and plants her foot to stand. The side on which the knee has been easier for Baby to bend is now the same side with which she plants her foot. If Baby hands-and-knees crawled with one knee up, the same up-knee leg will be the one she uses to plant her foot to push up to stand.

Please just observe and let her learn to stand her own way the first few days. When she has a feel for it, you can try the practice to help her tip to the less familiar side and plant the other foot—perhaps once a day for a couple of weeks until you see she can do it herself if she is inclined. Be sure to practice on a padded surface, as falling does happen. Falling is often fun for Baby, if it is not too startling and does not hurt.

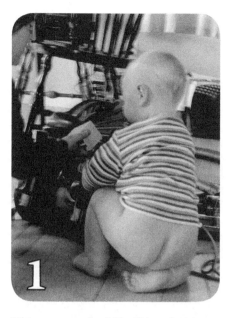

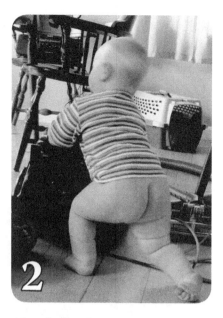

This ten-month-old half-kneel-sits on his more familiar side.

Here, he decides to stand up, pushing into his familiar foot.

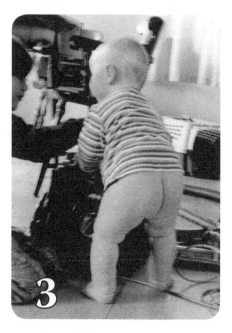

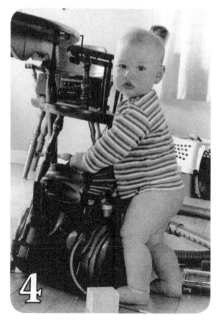

Next, he pulls his back leg forward, under his body, to standing.

He shifts to his familiar side again as he turns to the camera.

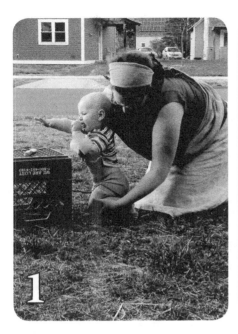

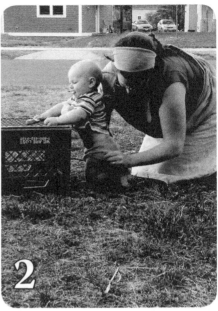

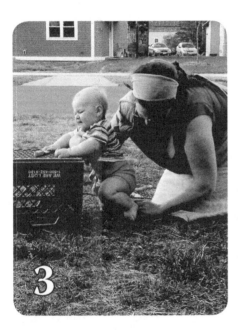

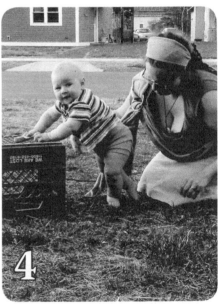

(P)ractice

Planting the Foot to Stand on the Less Familiar Side

1. Set up some kneeling play for Baby. Kneel nearby and be ready. This practice is done quickly.

2. Notice Baby's intention to stand from kneeling.

3. Just before she starts to move, tip her body slightly over her familiar side to help her opposite knee to pop up. Maintain your hand over Baby's shin until she lifts her less familiar leg and plants that foot on the ground. Wait until she begins to push up on that leg to stand, and then let go.

4. As soon as Baby's foot is on the ground, take your hand away. Let her discover the feeling of pushing with that foot and leg to move up.

Initially, Baby might not be able to push up fully on her less familiar leg. That is fine. Practice once a day, give or take, and you will see her strength grow in her weaker leg. With repetition, holding your hand over Baby's calf if she's kneeling and about to stand will be all that she needs to use her less familiar leg. Now it is more familiar!

Stairs can be a good place for this practice; be sure they are securely gated when not in use.

Getting Down From Standing

As soon as Baby pulls up to stand, it is time to teach her how to get down. We try to trigger her reflexes so she can go down with ease. Baby tends to quickly learn how to get down independently. Because she is a Baby, she does sometimes forget! She may be used to getting down from standing and then one day call or cry for your help. It is not easy being a baby at times.

(P)ractice

Unlock Baby's Waist To Drop Down

1. Hold Baby at the waist from behind her. Help her waist "fold" so that her behind reaches back as she drops to the floor. For many, this develops into intentional squatting.

2. With one hand on Baby's waist, gently tip her weight to one side. Use your other hand to bend the knee on the weight-free side. Now tip Baby's weight back over her bent-leg side and help her drop down. (This is how most adults get down).

3. Help Baby to bend at her waist, then bend her knees, easing her down into a squat. She may stay squatting, pop back up to standing, or drop to side-sitting.

Try It Yourself

Stand facing a sturdy support with both your hands resting on it, or down by your sides.

Now, gently lower yourself to the floor. What did you do?
- Lower your body into a squat?
- Lean to one side, bend the other leg, and lower it to the floor?
- Are your knees popping?
- Are you groaning?
- Did you inadvertently pull the chair down with you?
- Did your low-back feel vulnerable?
- Did you lower into a side-sitting, cross-legged, or another sitting position?
- Did you start to fall backward at any point and regain your balance?

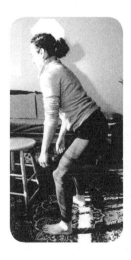 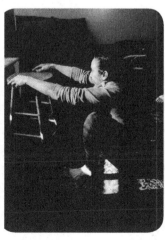 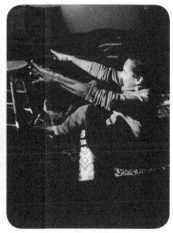

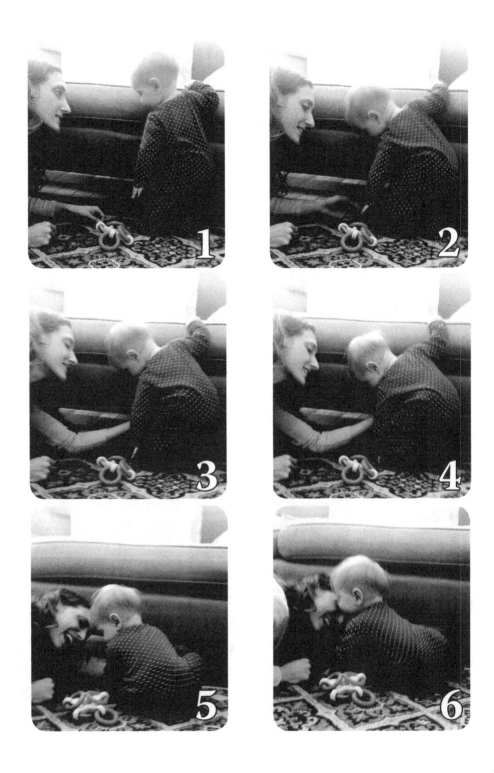

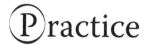ractice

Drop One Leg To Get Down

Soon Baby will learn to get safely down from standing by herself, rather than crying out for you to come help her.

In the following sequence an eight-month-old lowers herself down from standing to get a toy on the floor intentionally and accurately.

First, she sits down into her tail without even thinking about it. You can teach Baby how to get down from standing as soon as you see her starting to pull up. As a rule, help Baby get down from standing until she is expert at hands-and-knees crawling. Then she will be ready to stand naturally.

You don't need to prevent standing, but it is best not to encourage it. For the first few weeks when Baby pulls to stand, let her feel the position, then gently and firmly help her back to sitting using enticement or one of the physical practices described on the next page.

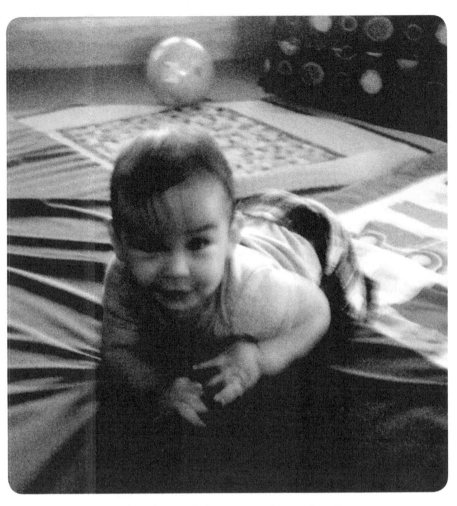

This seven-month-old understands "turn around to go down" and does so with a smile.

Climbing Up and Getting Back Down

Baby gets busy crawling on all fours. She may be able to stand; however, her momentum to go up might come before her momentum to step left or right. Baby has a deep drive to go up; she might climb a chair or climb up on the couch before she can side-step.

Whether she climbs and then side-steps or side-steps and then climbs, it is good to be prepared for Baby's climbing.

ⓟractice

'Turn Around To Go Down'

Teach your adventurous and sometimes fearless baby to turn around to go down, leading with her feet. The first few times, pick Baby up as you turn her, say "turn around to go down" and give a gentle pull on her feet to help her learn to drop her weight that way. You will be surprised how quickly Baby can learn to do this.

You might use a different choice of words. The essential part is to use the same words each time, and ask your mate and helpers if they could use these words too.

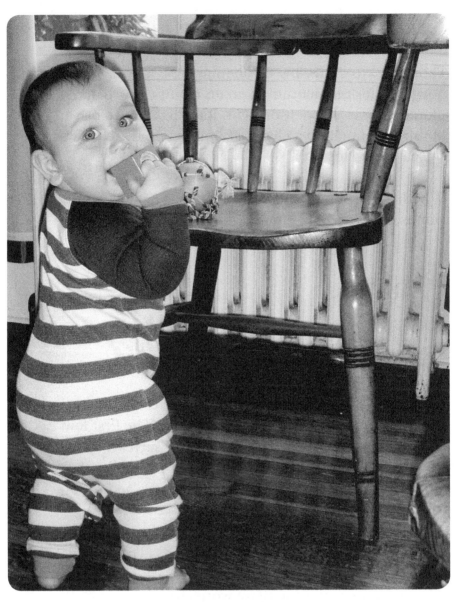

Eleven-month-old taking his first side-steps holding on with one hand.

Side-Stepping While Holding On

After learning to stand up and get back down, Baby begins to step to the side while holding onto a support. This is called side-stepping, or *cruising**. Side-stepping is a specific and important developmental movement milestone. Side-stepping strengthens hip muscles that complete the foundation for safe forward-walking. In Natural Movement Development, Baby side-steps for weeks, and then begins forward-walking when she's gained the strength to do so.

Baby usually steps to one side more easily than the other, just as she pushed with one side more than the other in belly-crawling. The same preference will show at every new stage.

Again, as with kneeling, nature offers an insurance policy in side-stepping for Baby to activate useful reflexes in her brain and body. This is especially valuable if she didn't belly-crawl when she was younger.

In belly-crawling, Baby shifts her pelvis to one side while reaching with her arm and pushes with her foot on the other side. In side-stepping, Baby reaches with her hand, tips her weight, and follows with her leg. For the next few weeks, give her many opportunities to do this playfully to both sides.

Baby tries to side-step using anything for support. She is determined and ingenious. Some safe supports are a low table without sharp corners, a sturdy push-toy, a sofa, or low chair.

This is similar to Baby learning to sit back from her hands-and-knees. Than, she sat to the familiar side, then sat to the other side, then found kneeling in the middle. Now, Baby steps to the familiar side, then learns to step to the less-familiar side, and then her brain and body put the sides together to make the whole, which is forward-walking.

Side-stepping is one of the reasons why it's important to refrain from "walking" your baby by upheld arms. In fact it is especially important because we get eager to see Baby walk and forget that side-stepping is the very thing that builds the strength for the walking we are waiting for. When we understand that side-stepping is an exciting skill for Bab,y we can enjoy watching how she grows it into walking.

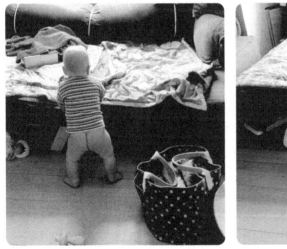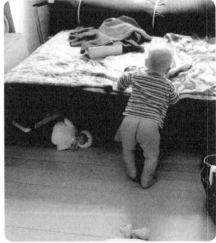

The family bed is great for side-stepping to one side and then the other.

“ As my son's first birthday approaches, I am savoring all of his movement stages that come before walking. Right now, my baby has a lot to see and do, and uses the method of movement that best suits his activity. He tries new things like holding two toys while still seeking support for standing, or side-stepping around a corner, first holding onto one piece of furniture and then another.

I can see his body becoming stronger and more sure of itself with each passing day. While I observe this progress, I am in no rush to hurry him through this phase of movement. He continues to use crawling as his main means of locomotion. He usually pulls up to standing or kneeling when he reaches his destination. After his curiosity is satisfied about something on the bookshelf, he drops back to sitting and turns to crawl across the floor to another toy. He still gets on his belly to retrieve something he wants from under a cabinet. He does all of these movements with such ease that it is hard to believe how challenging it was for him to learn each one! ”

A Mother

(P)ractice

Side-Stepping to Both Sides

- Make a space.
- Provide sturdy, kneeling-height furniture.
- Have incentives handy.

Once Baby has been standing, be sure to provide safe furniture to support her side-stepping. Observe which side she steps toward more easily. Let her practice in the easier direction for the first few days. Then put interesting things

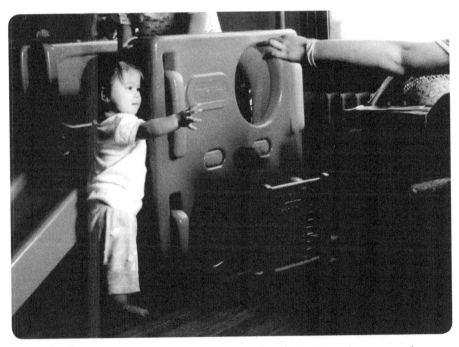

The yo-yo and its owner are the enticements that help this girl overcome her fear of falling as she shifts her weight to take her first side-steps.

at the other end of the supporting furniture and let her be enticed to step in that direction.

Practice using enticements to the less favored side when Baby is feeling playful, not tired. First, let Baby stand there and consider. If she takes a step and stops, bring her the object of her interest.

Play this way gently over time until she can step to both sides without hesitation. (The easier direction will be the same side on which Baby more easily bent her leg in belly-crawling).

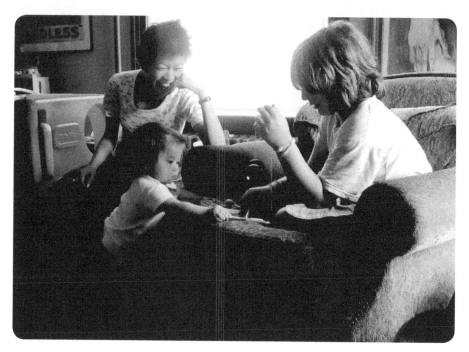

It was worth it!

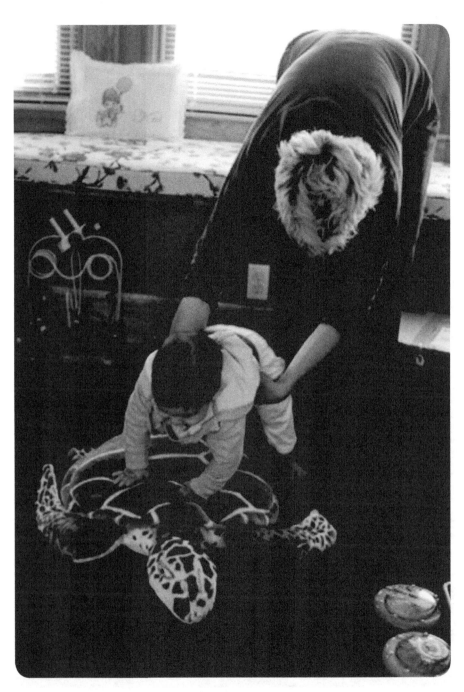

Arms-first is a natural way to put Baby down from your arms. This turtle is our arms-first friend. If you can, bend your knees a little and use your abs to protect your back as you lower Baby. Take care to stand up slowly.

Ⓟractice

Arms-First Baby Continues

If your back is strong enough, hold baby by the waist and put her down to her hands-and-knees. From there she can crawl, kneel, and knee-walk, or pop up to standing to toddle off, depending on her stage of movement.

Through the day, Baby often wants to be put down. Use these moments to lower her down, arms-first. This requires strength on your part. Check that your hands are not covering her arms so she can extend them to brace herself. These landings help her build necessary arm strength.

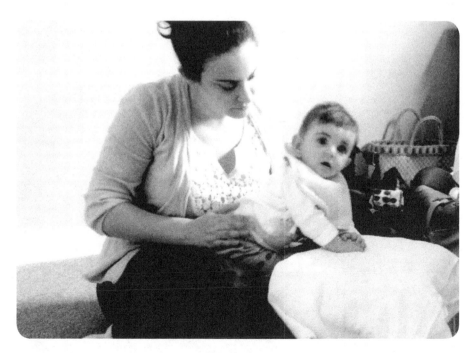

Mom helps Baby build arm strength while burping. Sometimes, this position gets the burp right out!

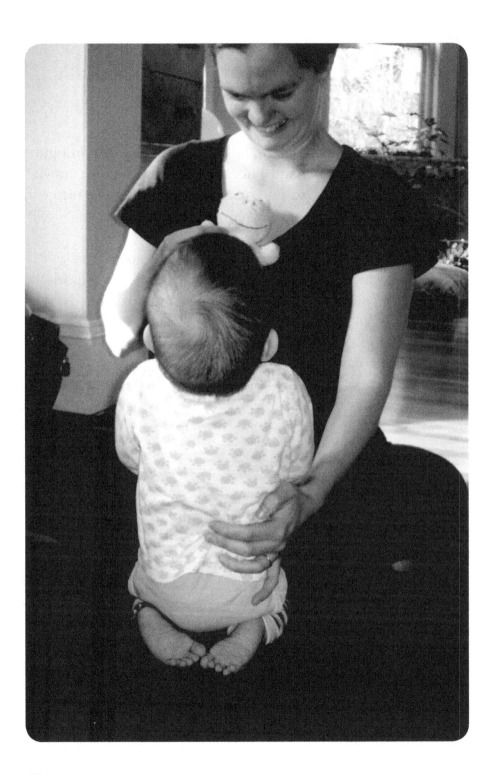

Natural Alternatives
to Prop-Standing

- Arms-first into hands-and-knees, or floor, as Baby chooses.

- Visiting at your lap in kneeling.

- Independent kneeling.

- Kneel-standing.

- Hands-and-knees positioning and play.

- Leaning and sitting.

- Swinging.

- Parent and Baby sit-dancing.

- Parent and Baby informal Yoga.

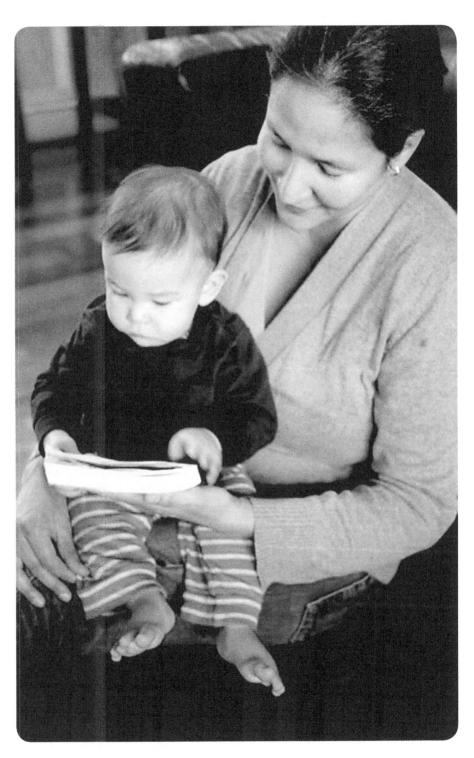

Taking Care Along the Way

Baby's transformation from someone who stays where you left her to someone who moves all over the place is indescribably miraculous! How could so much change happen so quickly? She wants to go everywhere, touch and hold and mouth everything. When she's awake, she's busy, busy. What joy! And sometimes a bit exhausting. Baby's attention shifts often, through the hour and the day.

As Baby is now on the go most of the time, her voracious appetite for life leading her everywhere, try to make note of when, and how, she rests. Can you find a way to have any of those *rest notes** in your routine together? Which do you both find relaxing, one at a time or in combination?

- Read together.

- Sing for Baby, or play Baby's favorite music.

* Dance, even if sitting.

- Lay Baby in the hammock, or lie together.

- Swing Baby on the swings.

- Walk indoors wearing baby.

- Push Baby in a stroller.

- Walk in nature wearing Baby.

- Side-by-side, focus when Baby focuses.

- Resting in a special cozy, partially concealed spot.

- Try a class such as Parent and Baby yoga.

Baby may have so much energy once she gets crawling that you are amazed by it.

Sometimes you may feel as if you cannot keep up with Baby. And why not? You have been parenting and losing sleep. She has been resting, eating, playing, and gaining strength.

Baby may have more endurance for a play session than you do. You might be surprised that this bigger version of Baby wants to be down on her tummy to move about. This is different from the Baby whom you carefully helped to tolerate TummyTime in the early weeks.

Now that Baby is often busy with toys, it helps to have a few buckets of toys that offer differing results.

I recommend toys without batteries in the first year if possible. This helps Baby to understand her own power without the added abstract kind of power that comes with batteries—something Baby cannot yet understand. However, a few of Baby's favorites toy may have batteries — somehow these get into your house — and these are sometimes helpful if you want to explore some flexion practice without Baby noticing, because her attention on her toy.

Toys that offer surprises (fun but not too startling), are often good helpers for Baby and you if you are going to do a little movement and bodywork practice. Examples include:

wind-up toys, rain sticks, a push toy that rolls across the floor, spinning mobiles, liquid motion toys, large and small soft balls, and containers full of similars such as a bucket of large pasta shapes or a basket full of easy-to-grasp blocks. Please see Appendix 3, pg. 351 for more suggestions.

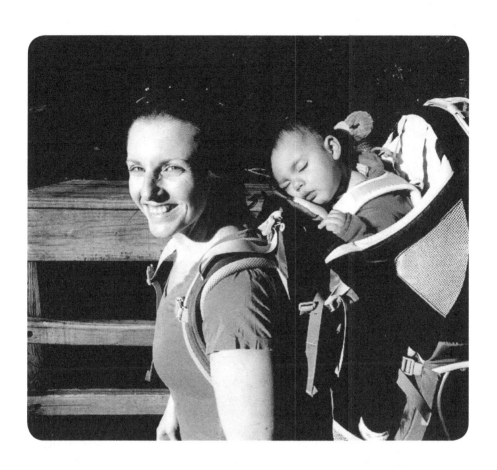

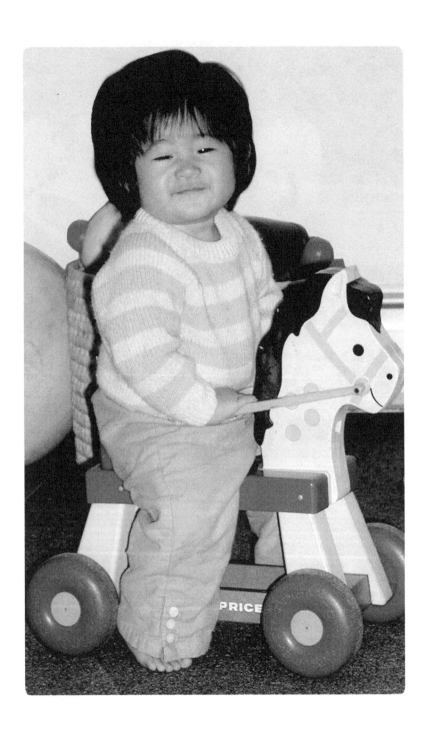

Standing *Leads to:*

- *dropping back down to crawl, then standing again.*

More Standing *Leads to:*

- *side-stepping.*
- *riding toys.*

Side-stepping and Stepping While Holding On with One Hand *Leads to:*

- *walking.*
- *toddling.*

Walking

Walking forward involves a weight shift, a small fall, and a regaining of balance on the other leg.

When Baby's arms swing freely, walking is an upright version of hands-and-knees crawling with all the weight in the spine and legs, and not in the arms, as in crawling; yet the rhythm of movement in the arms and legs is the same.

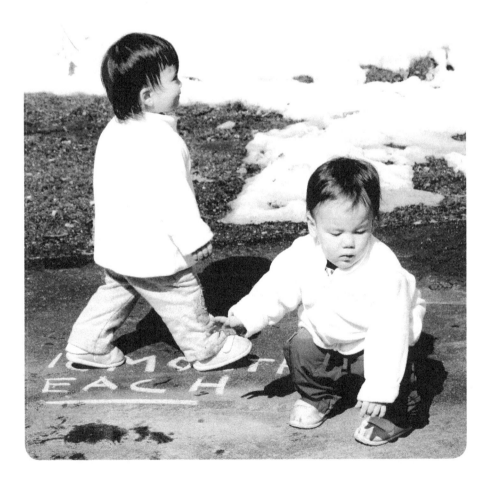

Walking *Leads to:*

- *toddling.*
- *running.*
- *climbing.*
- *driving toy vehicles.*
- *jumping.*
- *hopping.*
- *skipping.*

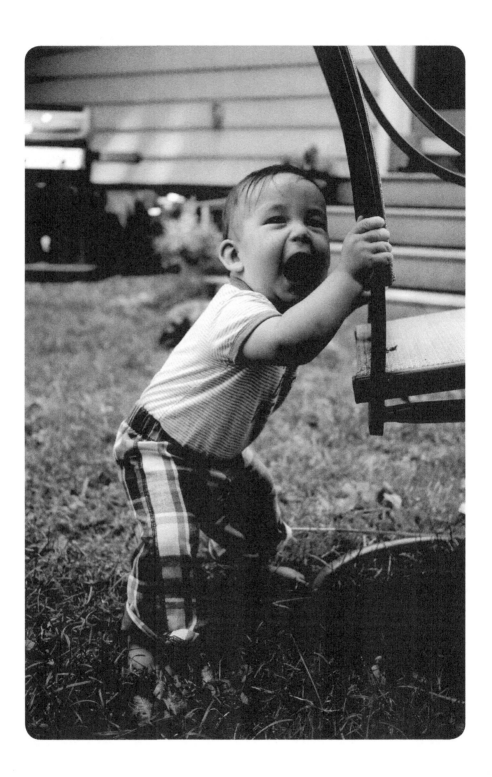

Summary

Congratulations! You've made it to the end of this book and through the first year, or more, of your beautiful new baby's life. No matter how Baby uniquely got walking, it has been a pleasure to be there on the way with you. Soon he will be running, jumping, making new chapters in the amazing journey you share as Baby continues to grow and bloom.

As parents and care providers, we can participate in the movement for sustainability. My point is that a sustainable lifestyle is one that includes the physical life of your Baby.

Sustainability can be applied to choices in every area of our lives. A way to live sustainably is to utilize and fertilize Baby's built-in natural resources as he grows. We do this by using less propping equipment and by letting Baby's movement and interests — and our playtime with Baby as we follow his lead — be our priorities.

Parenting with Natural Movement Development supports opportunities to resolve his startle responses, build his inner foundation, and grow naturally, from the floor up, free to move along his way. We bring our awareness and intuition, and we provide loving flexion and compression as his home base.

I hope this gives Baby and you a positive foundation, a sense of strength and resilience in relation to gravity, and the capacity to explore and to rest as you keep on growing and going.

We are all always on the way.

Appendix 1
Products Parents Ask About

Pacifier

How lucky is the child needing to suck who is given the pacifier when there is no breast, bottle, or finger to give! This is the individual choice of every family. Do try more than one brand, shape and size to see which Baby prefers, if any.

Nursing Pillow (e.g., Boppy®)

The nursing pillow is designed to increase comfort for Baby and parent when nursing. It might be used as a place to put Baby, but this is not the original purpose. Baby is meant to lie on her back without a pillow and on her side or tummy without a pillow. None of her reflexes are optimized when she lies on the pillow. It can be used for safety for Baby when needed, but it is not recommended as a propping tool for TummyTime.

Bolster

A bolster is not necessary for an infant, unless there are extenuating circumstances. If Baby is uncomfortable on her tummy, she needs very short visits there, with good company. The Bolster prevents her forearms from making contact with the floor. It is her own weight in the front of her forearms that activates the reflexes she needs to make her own strong triangle of support on the floor in TummyTime. The bolster actually *blocks the development of these reflexes*, making TummyTime harder.

Swing and Hammock

I recommend a swing for indoor support for Baby and you. Some can be hung from the ceiling, others stand alone. Swings, hammocks, and cradles offer Baby a chance to sit, lie flat, or only slightly elevated while rocking gently. She will like it even more if you place it where shadows play on the ceiling when she looks up. Or drape a piece of patterned fabric there for her to enjoy.

Jumper

When the jumper hangs low to the floor and allows Baby's feet to make contact with the floor, she will push and push. This pushing will overdevelop the thrusting reflexes in her legs. When this thrust is overactive, it is difficult for her to bend her legs at times, particularly on her tummy for belly-crawling. She pushes off from her feet repeatedly, before she knows how to roll or push back or belly-crawl forward. This actually makes the development of those skills more difficult. A baby who is often in the jumper, no matter how much she loves it, is also the same baby who "wants to stand all the time" and walks early without much time on the floor. This is not the end of the world, but it is easily avoided by choosing a safer piece of equipment for Baby to have soothing, moving time off your body, such as an indoor baby hammock, or automated cradle.

Shoes

Choose soft shoes for warmth and protection as long as Baby is not forward-walking. Comfortable sneakers are a great first shoe to try, after Baby is safely walking independently indoors.

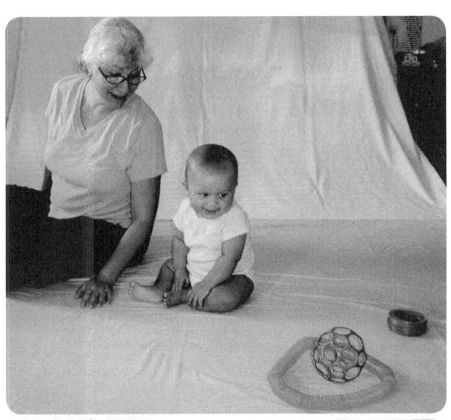

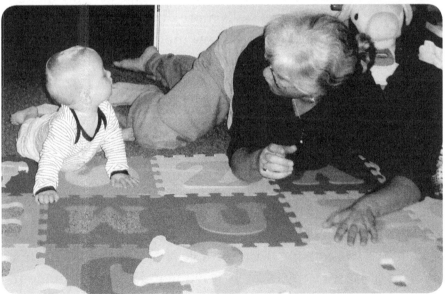

Appendix 2
Earliest Toys

- Double-sided baby mirror.

- Plain bracelets, pool or toss-rings, wooden rings.

- Simple, easy-to-grasp rattle.

- Simple, cozy stuffed-animal or doll.

- O-ball, various sizes (start small).

- Subtle, battery-free toys, such as a ball with a bell inside.

- Colorful interlocking foam floor tiles.

- Activity boards for floor-play, without batteries.

At first Baby doesn't want or need toys. He looks at your face and other faces, he notices light and dark, he watches things move. Baby gets interested in toys as his attention focuses outwardly more often. This happens early for some and later for others. Once he can, Baby often wants to mouth something for comfort and learning, such as while looking at a new face. This helps him stay calm as he takes in someone new, learning about them, and often breaking into a smile when he is done!

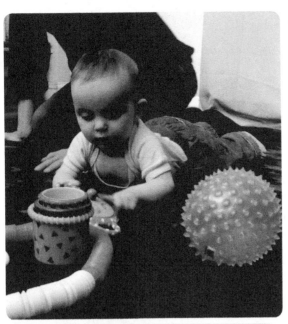

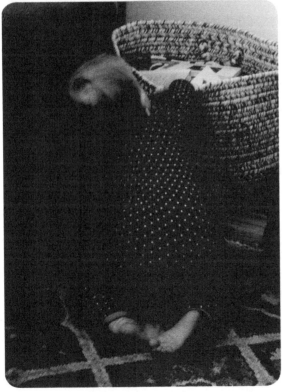

Appendix 3
Toys for Starting
To Get Around and Busy, Busy

- Simple wooden instruments.

- Buckets and baskets, some filled with books.

- A few stuffed animals, a favorite doll or blanket.

- Simple things to mouth.

- Something to spin.

- Something to sit in while it is spinning.

- Stable things to push.

- A firm table or stool to kneel at.

- Push-stick with bouncing balls at the end.

- Indoor plastic slide.

- Sturdy wooden push-toy with a lid that opens and closes.

- Collapsible stroller.

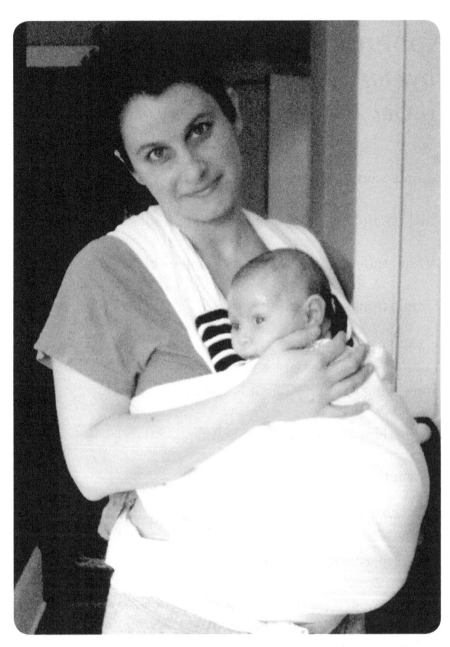

This three-week-old considers his world from a place of comfort.

Appendix 4
Gift Suggestions for New Parents

- Toys and equipment to support the practices in this book.

- TummyTime Station in a bag (a firm mat and a half-dozen colorful, soft quick-dry towels).

- Baby-wearing wraps.

- 2 three-pack Velcro swaddle wraps, smallest size and next size.

- 8 large organic towels: washed, folded, and stacked in a basket.

- Organic pajama sacks.

- 2 washable yoga mats: pre-washed.

- 4 ring-toss hoops or bracelets.

- Small and medium O-ball.

- Sturdy kneel-table.

- Absorbent blankets made specifically for TummyTime, padded blankets, available in cute designs.

- Set of large clear buckets with snap handles. Perhaps in one, a few infant toys, in another, swaddle wraps and a Moby, in the third some cardboard books.

- Comfortable rocker with footstool.

For a complete list, please visit www.amajoy.net and www.onthewaytowalking.com.

Appendix 5
How Propping Makes Natural Movement Development Difficult

- It inhibits the reflex responses that lead to rolling, crawling, and other movements.

- It prevents Baby from learning how to move from tummy to sitting, and from sitting to tummy. Continued prop-sitting blocks Baby's ability to move from sitting to hands-and-knees crawling.

- It increases Baby's leg thrusting. This makes it difficult for Baby to bend her knees naturally in order to feel comfortable in all the positions that might precede standing.

- It inhibits Baby's self-protective reflex responses from engaging. This weakens her ability to protect herself during movement and can have impact negatively on the development of her physical and psychological confidence.

- Frequently propped infants stand early and generally don't crawl. This can contribute to frequent falling, joint pain, learning issues, sensory sensitivities, and challenges with self-regulation.

- Generally, her ability to self-regulate while lying down is diminished if she is physically and emotionally used to being upright with her legs locked. It can be stressful for Baby, and you, if you do not provide the propping to which she has become accustomed.

Appendix 6
Common Propping Practices

• Placing Baby over a Boppy, or rolled towel for TummyTime.

• Placing Baby in a sitting position and encouraging her to stay there without support, by tightening her back muscles. Keeping Baby sitting with equipment such as a Bumbo chair.

• Holding Baby under her armpits to move or carry her.

• Sitting or standing Baby up from lying on her back by pulling her up with her hands. She keeps her body rigid and ends up standing on her toes on the floor or your lap.

• Holding Baby in a standing position with your hands around her waist, with her feet on you or the table or floor.

• Hanging Baby in a jumper or other device with a sling that runs between her legs so that she hangs by her crotch with no support under her bottom, her legs dangling.

• Hanging Baby in a jumper in which she repeatedly pushes off the floor with her feet.

• Holding Baby up in the air above your head with your hands around her as a frequent form of play or distraction.

• Walking behind Baby, holding her arms above her head and pulling some of her weight. She looks like she is walking, but she would fall if you let go.

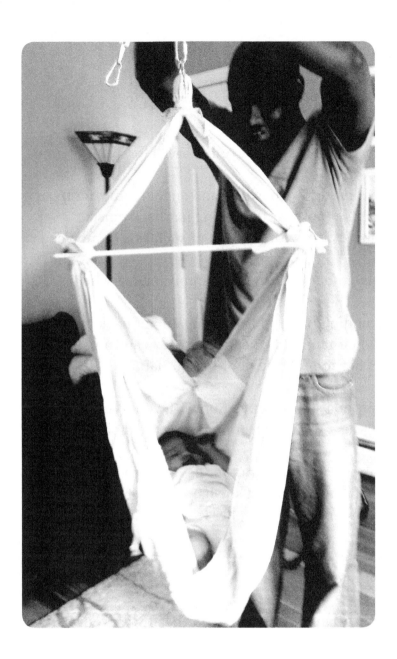

Appendix 7
Ways To Decrease Propping

• Regroup in Baby Ball after startle.

• Place Baby on her back, left, right, or tummy more often.

• Place Baby down from your embrace, arms-first to the floor or hip-first, to her side.

• Use floor-based activity centers, without batteries, and hang mobiles above floor-play space.

• Try wearing a sling, using an infant swing, or an indoor hammock. These can hang or have a floor base.

• Refrain from prop-sitting Baby; wait until she can push to sitting from rolling on her own.

• Limit prop-standing until baby can pull up to standing on her own. Even then it helps Baby to become strong and safe if you continue to place her down to hands-and-knees until she can walk smoothly.

• Play with Baby in side-lying, rolling, leaning, hands-and-knees, and kneeling. Try all of these yourself.

Observe your baby's body and movements, not only his facial expressions and utterances. Try to help him achieve his movement intentions. Observe what he can do himself. Offer small help in his hard spots and let him do the rest.

Appendix 8
Playing With the Senses

We find all kinds of ways to play with Baby, we try to notice what Baby likes, we pass along traditional songs, stories, games and recipes, all of which nourish Baby's senses.

This is a basic list of the senses. You might like to refer to it to make up games, including combining different senses in varying ways. We all have sensory preferences, and maybe some sensitivities. Explore together to find play that Baby and you both enjoy.

- Hearing: Snuggling, talking, cooing, singing, playing music, making music, humming, and goofing with language and sound, listening and uttering, call and response.

- Smelling: Milk or formula, the scent of parents and caretakers, food, and the environment. Babies recognize foods as being different than toys because of smell. Smell helps develop his sense of taste.

- Tasting: Milk or formula, foods, and things he puts in his mouth. Whenever Baby starts with solids, his senses of smell, taste, and sensation will guide what he does and doesn't like. You will know when he doesn't — you cannot miss the evidence.

- Seeing: Baby has heard and felt you, and experienced some changes in light and dark. When newly born, he turns towards the sounds of your voice. Baby sees light and dark, color, shape, and soon recognizes family faces.

- Feeling: Touch, weight, texture, and temperature. Baby knows exactly how you feel, and learns about much of his environment through touching with his hands, feet, and all his skin, as well as by feeling by mouthing. Giving and receiving sensation are both part of feeling.

- Moving: Baby moves *in utero* from the beginning. Movement is Baby's sense of self in space. He learns to move, and as he moves he encounters the world and learns. Baby loves to move. He wants to roll, spin, run, climb, and fly.

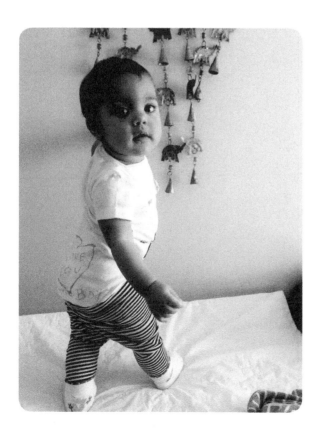

References

Chapter 1, pg. 9, Majnemer, A., & Barr, R. G. (2005). Influence of supine sleep positioning on early motor milestone acquisition. *Developmental Medicine & Child Neurology, 47*(6), 370-376. doi:10.1111/j.1469-8749.2005.tb01156.x

Chapter 5, pg. 137, American Academy of Pediatrics, www.aap.org "The American Academy of Pediatrics (AAP) released its recommendation in 1992 that infants be placed for sleep in a nonprone position." They also recommend Back to Sleep, Tummy to Play.

From the National Institute of Child Health and Human Development (NICHD) website- www.nichd.nih.gov/sts/Pages/default. aspx "Safe to Sleep® started in 1994 as the Back to Sleep campaign with the goal of educating parents, caregivers, and health care providers about ways to reduce the risk of SIDS."

Chapter 1, pg. 15. Chapter 3, pg. 92, Chutroo B., Jamrog, S. *Unpublished Manuscript*

Chapter 5, pg. 141, Majnemer, A., & Barr, R. G. (2005). Influence of supine sleep positioning on early motor milestone acquisition. *Developmental Medicine & Child Neurology, 47*(6), 370-376. doi:10.1111/j.1469-8749.2005.tb01156.x

Further Reading

Alexander, R., Boehme, R., & Cupps, B. (1993). *Normal Development of Functional Motor Skills: The First Year of Life*. Tucson, AZ: Therapy Skill Builders.

Ayres, A. J. (2005). *Sensory Integration and the Child* (25th Anniversary ed.). Los Angeles, CA: Western Psychological Services .

Bainbridge Cohen, B. (1994). *Sensing, Feeling, and Action: The Experiential Anatomy of Body-Mind Centering*. Northampton, MA: Contact Editions.

Bauer, I. (2001). *Diaper Free: The Gentle Wisdom of Natural Infant Hygiene*. United Kingdom: Plume.

Borgenicht L, M.D. and Borgenicht, J. (2012). *The Baby Owner's Manual: Operating Instructions, Trouble-Shooting Tips, and Advice on First-Year Maintenance* (2nd ed.). Philadelphia, PA: Quirk Books

Bryt, M., (1998). *Baby Love: A tradition of calm parenting*. New York, NY: Dell Publishing.

Goddard Blythe, S. (2005). *Reflexes, Learning and Behavior*. UK: INPP Ltd.

Hannaford, C. Ph.D. (2005). *Smart Moves: Why Learning Is Ñot All in Your Head*. Salt Lake City, Utah: Great River Books.

Hartley, L., (1995). *Wisdom of the Moving Body*. Berkeley, CA: North Atlantic Books.

Karp, H. (2002) *The Happiest Baby on the Block.* New York, NY: Dell Publishing

Leach, P. (1997). *Your Baby and Child: From Birth to Age Five* (3rd ed.). New York: Alfred A. Knopf.

Majnemer, A., & Barr, R. G. (2005). *Developmental Medicine & Child Neurology, 47*(6), 370-376. doi:10.1111/j.1469-8749.2005.tb01156.x

McCormack, D., Perrin, K. (1997). *Spatial, Temporal, and Physical Analysis of Motor Control.* San Antonio, TX: Therapy Skill Builders

Murphy, J. (2000) *Baby's First Year.* Tuscon, AZ: Fisher Books

Nilsson, L. (1990). *A Child Is Born* (C. James, Trans.). New York, NY: Dell Publishing.

Payne, J. K. (2010). *Simplicity Parenting.* New York, NY: Ballantine Books.

Schoenwolf, G., Bleyl, S., Brauer, P., & Francis-West, P. (2009). *Larsen's Human Embryology* (4th ed.). United Kingdom: Churchill Livingston.

Shelnov, S., American Academy of Pediatrics. (1998) *The Complete and Authoritative Guide: Caring For Your Baby and Young Child* (Rev. ed). New York, NY: Bantam Books

Solter, A. (2001). *Aware Baby* (Rev. ed.). Goleta, CA: Shining Star Press.

Swain, J. (Circa 2010). *Emmi Pikler's Trust in the Wise Infant*

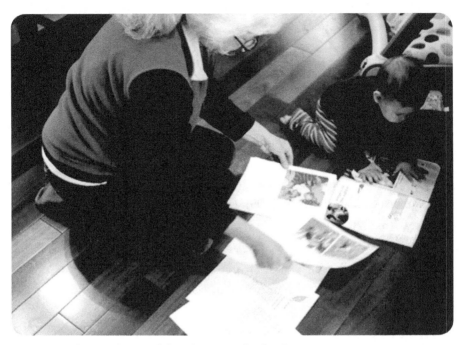

Lenore working with one of the editors on this book.

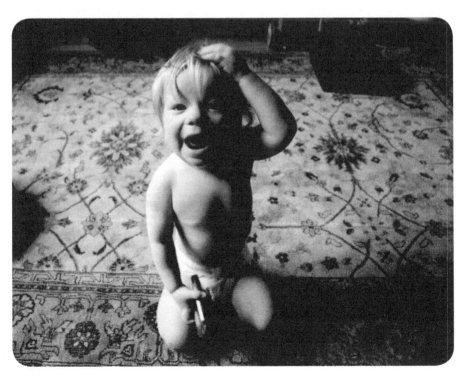

Glossary

Airplane Reflex (Landau reflex) - full extension of the spine, arms, and legs while on the tummy.

All Terrain Baby - expertise in crawling over variable and unpredictable surfaces.

Baby Ball - a core practice in Natural Movement Development. It supports all the rest of the practices with parents providing Baby with *flexion* and *compression*. See C-curve.

Back to Sleep Campaign - initiated in 1994 by the AMA and adopted by several western countries; instruction to parents to sleep babies exclusively on their backs for the prevention of SIDS.

Bear-Standing - a developmental movement when Baby stands with his weight on his hands and on his feet, with his bottom up and his head down.

Bear-Walking - when a baby is able to step in *Bear-Standing* (see above).

Belly-Crawling - a baby's first independent movement, which marks the increasing desire to explore and the beginning of a new phase.

C-Curve - a natural inward curving of the spine, which remains a resting place throughout childhood, reminiscent of the fetal position.

Commando Crawling or Pre-Crawling - Crawling while on the belly, by pulling the body forward one arm at a time along the floor, without using the legs to push.

Compression - holding someone's body with gentle, firm, surrounding pressure.

Connective Tissue Impression - the position most familiar to a baby's body, based on how they were compressed *in utero.*

Crab-Crawling - hands-and-knees crawling with one knee up. Baby moves on 2 hands, one knee, and one foot (with that knee not touching the ground).

Craniosacral Therapy - a gentle, effective hands-on method of healing for infants, children, and adults. *(upledger.com)*

Crawling - academic description of moving forward along the belly, but commonly used to mean moving on hands-and-knees.

Creeping - academic description of crawling on hands-and-knees.

Cross-Crawling - a term for hands-and-knees crawling.

Developmental Movement - universal movements that all infants go through to a greater or lesser degree.

Extension - thrusting or arching movements that strengthen the extensor muscles on the back.

Feldenkrais - a method of healing using movement and touch developed by Moshe Feldenkrais. (*Feldenkrais.com*)

Fine Motor Development - skills and activities that use the hands and fingers, feet and toes.

Flexion - an essential tool for helping Baby return to his original feelings of contained comfort.

Flexion Teacher – a physical part of parenting, including holding one's child in a C-curve position with compression.

Flexion-to-Flexion Reflex - a lifelong reflex in which the baby yields into the adult, and the adult folds around the baby.

Gross Motor Development - skills using the larger movements Baby makes with arms, legs, feet, and entire body.

Hand-to-Mouth Reflex - this reflex works together with rooting and sucking reflexes. This reflex may be set off by either stroking your baby's cheek or the palm of her hand. The stroking causes your baby to root, her arm to flex, and to bring her hand to her mouth.

High Tone - tissues at rest, including muscles, organs, and nerves, are less able to release into gravity.

Infant Developmental Movement Education - a two-year training offered by the school for Body-Mind Centering. Students learn to recognize movement patterns and to interact with infants for a positive effect on development. *(bmcassoc.org)*

Knee-Walking - walking on bent legs with the body weight in the knees and forelegs.

Landau Reflex - full extension of the spine, arms, and legs while on the tummy.

Low Brain - the part of the brain that controls reflexes, or "random movements."

Low Tone - tissues at rest, including muscles, organs, and nerves, are less able to move away from gravity.

Moro Reflex - an infantile reflex normally present in all infants/newborns up to 4 or 5 months of age as a response to sudden loss of support, when the infant feels as if it is falling. It involves three distinct components:
1. stimulus position
2. spreading out the arms and legs (abduction and extension)
3. pulling in the arms and legs (adduction and flexion).

Narrow the Base- a manual technique in NMD to bring Baby's legs under her pelvis when she is kneeling for increased stability and engagement of reflex support.

Natural Movement Development (NMD)- infant movement development that supports parents to let Baby learn to move from the floor upward, with minimal propping.

Neonatal Startle - earliest startle, involving the whole body.

Protective Extension - extending the arms to protect the head when feeling oneself falling.

Propping - upright positioning of Baby while held by an adult or equipment. These are positions in which she doesn't yet have the skills to protect herself if she tips or falls.

Reflexes -part of a web of internal and external responses, reflexes are part of our basic movements and perceptions, and how these work together. They usually occur outside of awareness. A newborn Baby's movements are due in large part to reflex responses to his internal and outer environment.

Rest Notes - little moments when Baby is still or quiet when parent/caregiver also rests.

Safe Small Fall - the shortest, safest fall, later resulting in Baby being able to do the same movement without falling.

Self-Regulation - the ability to respond to one's inner cues for digestion, rest, recuperation, etc.

Startle Reflex - see Moro Reflex.

Sucking Reflex - response to sensations on the skin around the lips, directly on the lips, tongue, and insides of the mouth, that cause Baby to suck and swallow.

Thrusting Reflex - a response to movement, position or other stimulus, in which Baby intensifies his extension muscles to lock both legs in straight pushing with his knees locked.

Tip Him Up - using the least amount of touch possible to help Baby complete his movement from lying to sitting without falling backward in the process.

Acknowledgements

Heartfelt thanks to the families who allowed us to print their images. No babies, no book!

Photo Credits: Sarah Buttenwieser, Can Stock Photo Inc., Barbara Chutroo, Jahara Sara Conz, Mindy Couture, Elizabeth Cordova, Belinda Del Pesco, Allan Doe, Emily and Shir Feit, Amy Gilburg, Lenore Grubinger, Cody Hindes, Sarah Hougen, Brian and Jennifer Hydefrost, Alexis Major Jameson, Neal Jameson, Laurie Johnson, Jano Julmy, Joanna Krueger, Douglas MacKenzie, Marta Martinez, Sondra Peron, Kipngetich Rutto, Karen Sullivan, and Naho Tanamura-Green.

Illustration Credit: Karen Kuchar, pg. 5, used with permission.

Huge gratitude to:
— Gordon Thorne, Anne Woodhull, and Ann Thompson of fiscal sponsor Available Potential Enterprises (A.P.E.). for staying behind this project for the long haul. We could not have done it without you!
— the Solidago Foundation for their generous support early on.
— the editors, for their excellence, and for bartering through Valley Time Trade: Hazel Adolphson, Alexis Major Jameson, Chris Rohmann, and Robin Thompson. Jane Johnson, your kindness and fastidious work over innumerable hours brought us to the finish.
— the awesome people who generously gave every kind of support: Lorraine Barbieri, Hosea Baskin, Catherine Burns, Sarah Werthan Buttenwieser, Barbara Chutroo, Bob and Barbara Dell, Tracey Devlin, Sam Doe, Emily Feit, Shir Feit, Jen Gallant, Michelle Gay, Ari Greenberg, Eva Grubinger, Vern Grubinger, Louisa Hall, Jennifer Hydefrost, Phyllis Krechevsky, Jim Levey, Donald Lewis, Gwen McClellan, Christine Olson, Eliza Parker, Sarah Pirtle, Marianne Simon, Steve Strimer, Linda Tumbarello, Maiken Wallinger, and Sarah Willey.

— Bonnie Bainbridge Cohen, love and gratitude, as ever and ever.

— Jahara Sara Conz, for your special spirit, talent, and commitment. I owe this book to your help. Shine on!

— Elizabeth Cordova, for being this book's *Madrina;* your generosity and faith made it possible.

— Belinda Del Pesco, for always being taller and smarter than me, for gently and generously showing me the way, and for filling the world with beauty.

— Cody Hindes, for being in the right place at the right time, and for linking us to the world.

— Phyllis Krechevsky, Amajoy Angel, for friendship over the whole way. You have been there since before we started and will be there after we are done, so we'll never be done.

— Anna Penenberg, for reading and wisely commenting on 1,001 revisions, and for cheering us up and on.

— Allan Doe, thank you for being you, and for making dreams come true.

Please forgive any omissions, they are the unintentional fault of the author.

In grateful memory of Suzanne Green River, founder of Global Somatics. She gave her encouragement and ideas passionately for this book, from the beginning in 2000 until shortly before her death in February, 2014.

INDEX

Focus Points

Natural Alternatives To

Natural Movement in Pictures   33-45

Practices

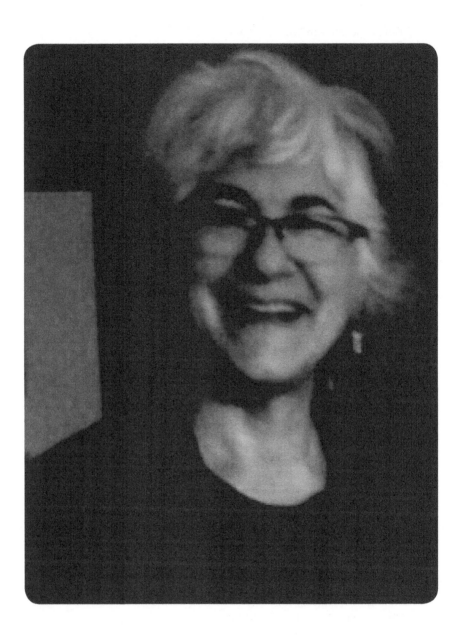

On the Way to Walking

About the Author

Lenore Grubinger is the founder and director of Amajoy Developmental Movement and Bodywork, in Florence, Massachusetts. She has conducted private practice for over thirty-five years, and leads workshops for parents and family-serving professionals in the US and abroad.

Ms. Grubinger earned her BA in 1984 from the University of Massachusetts, Amherst, in Somatic Studies.

Ms. Grubinger earned Practitioner and Teacher certification in Body-Mind Centering® (BMC) in 1986. She taught periodically over thirty years at the School for Body-Mind Centering (SBMC), in the certification and teacher certification programs.

She completed advanced training in CranialSacral Therapy with Dr. John Upledger in 1988. Additionally Ms. Grubinger trained in Neurodevelopmental Therapy with Sara White.

Ms. Grubinger was curriculum director of Developmental Movement and Learning, an educational non-profit, from 2001- 2004.

A member of the International Somatic Movement Education and Therapy Association (ISMETA), Lenore is a Registered Somatic Movement Therapist (RSMT).

A co-developer of the Infant Developmental Movement Education (IDME) program of the SBMC, Ms. Grubinger taught in the IDME program from 2000 though 2009.

Made in the USA
Monee, IL
08 January 2023

24813016R00213